Reducing the Symptoms of Alzheimer's Disease and Other Dementias

Reducing the Symptoms of ALZHEIMER'S DISEASE and Other DEMENTIAS

A Guide to Personal Cognitive Rehabilitation Techniques

JACKIE POOL

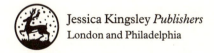

Jessica Kingsley *Publishers*
London and Philadelphia

The information contained in this book is not intended to replace the services of trained medical professionals or to be a substitute for medical advice. You are advised to consult a doctor on any matters relating to your health, and in particular on any matters that may require diagnosis or medical attention.

First published in 2019
by Jessica Kingsley Publishers
73 Collier Street
London N1 9BE, UK
and
400 Market Street, Suite 400
Philadelphia, PA 19106, USA

www.jkp.com

Library of Congress Cataloging in Publication Data
A CIP catalog record for this book is available from the Library of Congress

British Library Cataloguing in Publication Data
A CIP catalogue record for this book is available from the British Library

ISBN 978 1 78592 578 8
eISBN 978 1 78450 992 7

Printed and bound in Great Britain

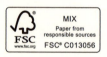

Contents

Chapter 1

My 40 Year Journey with Dementia

When I was a child, my Gran had dementia. Only we didn't know it was called that at the time. I think we thought of it as her having 'gone senile'. My parents, my sister and I could see she was acting 'strangely' and to be honest, at times we were not as supportive as we could have been. You could say that we didn't know any differently – there was no information, help or support and we simply followed the lead of the staff in the care home where Gran moved to live. Hindsight is always a wonderful thing, as they say, and I wish I had known then what I know now. Gran would certainly have had a much better experience, at least from her family members.

Moving forwards to my early twenties, I began my career in dementia as an occupational therapy assistant in a hospital in the North-West of England. This was in the 1980s when hospital services were known as 'psycho-geriatrics', and the building I worked in had previously been a workhouse for the poor and destitute. The belief at that time was that Alzheimer's disease was the main cause of the dementia and, as we didn't know the cause of Alzheimer's disease, there was nothing we could do apart from keep the patient clean, safe and occupied.

Anti-dementia medication had not arrived at that point and patients were routinely given anti-psychotic medication to address any behaviours that were thought to be a challenge. Care was task- and ward routine-driven and we had no idea of supporting patients to actually improve in cognition and function.

I shudder to think now that I almost didn't embark on my career in dementia care, so put off was I by my very first experience on that ward. I had arrived just when the nurses were all having their break. As I entered the day room, I saw a circle of large chairs containing elderly ladies all facing each other. Some were slumped with their eyes closed, some were watching with interest and several were shouting and waving their arms around. When I went to the first lady, who seemed the most distressed, she grabbed my arm and urgently said 'toilet!' The message was clear and I went to ask the nurses for guidance. They were seated at a table at the other end of the room and one nurse told me wearily that it wasn't time for doing the toilet round yet and that it would be carried out after they had finished their break. This duly happened and the experience was shocking. A bin bag was placed in the centre of the circle of chairs and then each lady had an incontinence pad removed, this was put in the bin bag and a new pad was placed on the chair. Each lady was wearing a similar cotton nightdress with a split up the back to make the task easier.

My gut feeling was that this was wrong – there was no sense of dignity or of humanity – and although the nurses were not intentionally unkind I felt that each lady had been dehumanised: treated as an object rather than a person. But, as the newest member of staff I assumed that the others knew best so I tried to fit in with their way of working. My role that first day was to entertain the group and I was asked to play a balloon game with the ladies, batting it to each of them to get a response. I went home in tears wondering what sort of work this would be. I kept going though and I soon began to connect with each of the ladies and to form relationships with them. As I became more involved I witnessed their individuality, of course, and I saw that each lady fluctuated in her abilities as well as in her struggles. I became convinced that there had to be more to living with dementia than 'balloons and incontinence pads' and that there must be more that we could do to enable the potential for those abilities to occur.

I decided to enrol to train as an occupational therapist (OT).

Three years later I started work as a newly qualified OT in North Wales at another older people's mental health services hospital. As you can see, the language for users of these services had begun to change to a more positive tone. And I was very fortunate in the support I had from my manager and from the consultant psychiatrist who actively encouraged my ongoing learning and development and who fostered my enthusiasm for improving the lives of people with dementia and their families.

At this time, in the early 1990s I began to read the work of Professor Tom Kitwood, a psychologist working with Bradford University. His 1990 paper, 'The dialectics of dementia: with particular reference to Alzheimer's disease', and his proposal for understanding dementia by applying a more holistic viewpoint than purely the neurological condition was groundbreaking and an eye-opener. I will explain more about Tom's application of a person-centred approach in Chapter 2. This new approach in dementia care gave hope and purpose to both academics and practitioners – 'at last there is something that we can do' was heard at many conferences and seminars in those early days as a solution to the 'no known cause therefore no cure' dominant medical approach. Much of what Tom said resonated with my own findings with my patients and I was very excited by this emerging framework for understanding and supporting people who are living with dementia. However, I was concerned that the risk was that 'the baby would be thrown out with the bath water' (so to speak) and that the focus on the social model would eclipse the medical one and lead us to ignore the cognitive difficulties that people with dementia experience. I wanted to go further than just support people to live well with their dementia. I wanted to address those cognitive difficulties so that people could improve in their function. I had already seen this happen with my patients when I focused on their specific problems and I wanted to learn more and formalise my approach.

So I wrote to Tom Kitwood to discuss my concerns about losing the focus on cognition and that was the start of an eight-year relationship during which we worked together, discussed, debated and shared ideas. It was because of him that I began to develop my thinking about systematically working to improve cognition and function and it was Tom that first encouraged me to write a book about this as part of the Bradford University Dementia Group Good Practice Guide series. However, my thinking took me in a slightly different direction from a purely 'how to' manual and led me to develop the Pool Activity Level (PAL) Instrument as a practical resource for understanding the levels of ability of people with dementia. We will explore the use of the PAL Instrument later, but it is worth mentioning now that it was during a discussion about the development of the PAL Instrument with Tom that the word 'rementia' was first raised in connection with my work. I was explaining to him how it is possible to determine the cognitive function ability of an individual and then to probe for a higher level of performance. He exclaimed: 'But that is rementia, Jackie!'

Tom had only just begun to think about this phenomenon in a paper he had published in 1989 but more was to follow and we will look at the ideas behind this when we get to Chapter 3.

Tom Kitwood was a pioneer in the field of dementia care. He was the author of numerous publications on dementia and he won the Age Concern 'book of the year' award for *Dementia Reconsidered* (1997). He developed innovative research projects and training courses, challenging the non-person-centred culture of care. In September 1998 he gained a personal chair from Bradford University and was appointed the Alois Alzheimer Professor of Psychogerontology. Sadly and unexpectedly, he died later that same year. Tom was a great communicator and well known for his charisma in delivering courses, presentations, conferences and seminars. He was an inspiration to many people world-wide, including me.

During the eight years of our friendship I had moved from working in a hospital setting to working in the South of England with a county council as an advisor to their care homes. My role was to work with residents with dementia and to support their care workers, but I became frustrated by the red tape and rules that prevented me from using the knowledge and practising the skills that I had developed. So, in 1995 I decided to set up my own consultancy for individuals with dementia. I regularly wrote and published my findings and because of this, I was frequently invited to talk about my work at conferences. From there, care providers asked me to lead some training for them and my business quickly grew from a one-woman consultancy to a UK-wide and international training and consultancy service to hospitals, care homes and other dementia care providers.

In 2009, I sat on the National Dementia Strategy external reference group, contributing to the shaping of our current framework for dementia care across all services and to the development of our first national dementia care qualification. In 2010, I was asked to write the Skills for Care Qualifications and Credit Framework for dementia.

It was about then that my mum developed dementia. Although looking back, she probably had the symptoms much sooner. She had motor neurone disease and her needs were complex. However, the experience of dementia for her was not all bad and in many ways she became a more free spirit than she ever was prior to her cognitive impairments. I felt fortunate to be able to use my knowledge to help Mum during the stages of her own journey. Sometimes I felt I had to battle with the services to get Mum the support that I knew would benefit her and, of course, I learned at firsthand what it is like to be a carer. There were difficult times, but there was also great fun. In September 2013 Mum died well with the condition.

During this period, as well as continuing to deliver dementia care training and developing resources for care providers, I was also invited to join a major research programme: the GREAT study (Goal-oriented cognitive Rehabilitation in Early-stage Alzheimer's disease: multi-centre single-blind randomised controlled Trial). The study aimed to find out whether cognitive rehabilitation is beneficial for people for people with dementia. The trial began in October 2012 and ended in December 2016. It took place in eight research centres across England and Wales, and in total there were 480 trial participants. My role as part of the Trial Management Group was to train and supervise the therapists in their delivery of cognitive rehabilitation.

As I write this we are now starting on the next phase of the GREAT study. This time it is a three-year project, from 2018– 2021, funded by the Alzheimer's Society. The title of the study is: 'Maintaining independence in Alzheimer's and related dementias through Goal-oriented cognitive REhAbiliTation: Implementation into Practice (GREAT-iP)'. In this study we will be beginning the process of enabling health and social care services to offer cognitive rehabilitation, adapting the interventions to real-life practice

I will be describing the rehabilitation approaches and how you can build them into a self-help programme in Chapter 6.

So, I have described my journey with dementia over 40 years, during which I have: developed clinical reasoning and practice skills; delivered hundreds of training courses to thousands of care workers; created resources that are used around the world to support dementia care development; spoken at national and international conferences; contributed to Government strategies; worked as a Dementia Ambassador, a Dementia Friend Champion and as a member of the Dementia Action Alliance. In fact, I have dedicated my life to trying to improve the lives of people with dementia.

Hence this book. I don't want my learning to go to waste when I end my professional career. I am conscious that I am now discussing pension plans with my husband and that I have car insurance with SAGA. It is time for me to make plans for ensuring what I have learned is not lost and that it gets to the people who would benefit the most. This, of course, is those who are living with dementia – the individual and their family and friends. While I know that health and social care professionals will also be interested in the content of this book, I also know that some aspects may be dismissed by them as not valid because not enough statistical data is available. Even so, the lived experience of dementia continues relentlessly for many and they haven't got time to wait for the research programmes. This book is therefore designed for those individuals who want to support others and for those who want to take matters into their own hands with a Rementia Plan for improving their experience by reducing the symptoms of dementia.

A word of caution, this is not a book claiming to have found a 'cure' for the neurological conditions that contribute to dementia. It is a framework for addressing and reversing the symptoms associated with the neurological conditions. So, Alzheimer's disease, vascular disease, Parkinson's disease, Lewy body disease, motor neurone disease, etc. may still be present but the individual may no longer have the symptoms, have fewer symptoms or have less disabling or distressing symptoms.

The approaches can be used by individuals at all levels of ability and the Rementia Plan in the final chapter will show you how. Talk of stages and particularly 'end-stage' leads us down No Hope Avenue and creates a self-fulfilling prophecy that individuals will spiral inevitably downwards. This does not fit with my experience that it is possible to support people at all levels of ability to live well at that level or higher. I am not suggesting that we can reverse the symptoms all the way back to when the person did not have the neurological condition, but I am going to show you how it is possible to find some degree of improvement or, at the least, to maintain the person's level of ability and to slow down the rate of progression of the symptoms of dementia.

The emotional impact of living with dementia when relationships are affected and communication is undermining cannot be ignored. In Chapter 4, I will be showing you how, by understanding the chemical reaction that takes place during interactions with each other, we can reduce or even prevent some of the symptoms of dementia.

Not all of the findings offered in this book are the results of independent, fully researched and documented, double-blind clinical studies, but that does not mean that there is no documented source. You will find all the references to articles and books by leading thinkers, academics and clinicians in the field in the References and Reading List at the end of this book.

This is particularly relevant when you get to Chapter 5 as the information about diet and nutritional supplements challenges the current health establishment orthodoxies. Having said that, even as I write this, there is a dawning realisation among health researchers that the dietary advice we have been fed for 40 years by our UK Government and by the US Government lacks proper evidence to support it. There is strong evidence emerging from reputable sources such as the University of the West of Scotland and the *British Medical Journal* that some of those orthodoxies may be responsible for obesity, diabetes and dementia. Indeed, some are now calling Alzheimer's disease 'Type 3 Diabetes' and the proposal is that there is a link between what we eat and our brain function. If you think about it, why wouldn't there be? We understand that what we put into our bodies affects our other organs and body system; why should it not also affect our brain?

It will be interesting to see where these findings will take us but meanwhile, for this book, I am drawing on the emerging research to propose that we should be very aware of the healthy heart equals healthy brain theory. In Chapter 5 I will set out the current thinking about diet for you so that you can make up your own mind and decide for yourself if you want to address this as part of your Rementia Plan.

In addition to covering diet, I will also be describing the effects of malnutrition and dehydration and how these conditions can cause the symptoms of dementia in any individual. On top of that, people who already have some degree of cognitive impairment are at higher risk of becoming malnourished and dehydrated, bringing with it a downward spiral into further dementia. I will explain the reasons why people with dementia are at such risk and how this can be prevented or reversed.

I believe that a healthy body and a healthy mind results in a healthier brain. To fight dementia and achieve rementia requires a multi-therapeutic approach that addresses every aspect for a healthy body, mind and brain.

Please do read this book and the additional reading with an open mind and, if you do embark on the suggested Rementia Plan, keep in touch and let me know how you get on. That way we can build data to develop our learning further and so help others too.

Chapter 2

What Dementia Is and Isn't

Many people think that they know what the word 'dementia' means, but often the cause of dementia and the symptoms of dementia are thought to be one and the same. The dictionary definition of dementia describes a person who is 'out of his mind', but even this is misleading as we really need to understand more about mind, cognition and memory to be able to understand what is happening when someone has dementia. Contrary to popular belief, dementia is not in itself a medical diagnosis. The neurological condition which is causing the individual to experience dementia should be the actual diagnosis: Alzheimer's disease, vascular disease, etc.

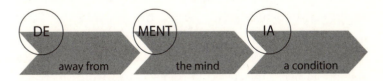

Myth: People with dementia don't know what they like, need or want.

Myth: People with dementia can't learn new things.

Myth: People with dementia revert to being children.

Myth: Dementia is a normal consequence of ageing.

Myth: If you get dementia, nothing can be done about it.

Myth: Alzheimer's disease and dementia are the same thing.

A very common question that I am asked is: 'Are Alzheimer's disease and dementia the same thing?' The Alzheimer's Society explains that the word dementia describes a set of symptoms that may include memory loss and difficulties with thinking, problem-solving or language. These changes are often small to start with, but for someone to be viewed as having dementia they have become severe enough to affect daily life.

It goes on to explain that the symptoms of dementia arise when the brain is damaged by diseases, such as Alzheimer's disease or blood vessel (vascular) disease. Alzheimer's disease is the most common cause of dementia, but not all dementia is due to Alzheimer's. The specific symptoms that someone with dementia experiences will depend on the parts of the brain that are damaged.

So, we can clearly see that from this explanation that dementia and Alzheimer's disease are not the same. Dementia is the group name for the symptoms. Alzheimer's disease is the name of one of the causes of those symptoms.

I think it helps to understand this by using a physical analogy: the common cold. We use this umbrella term as a quick way of describing a set of symptoms; a headache, sore throat, sneezes, cough, temperature. But these symptoms come from being infected by a rhinovirus, of which there are 99 recognised types.

Likewise, there are as many as 50 known causes of dementia, but most of these causes are very rare. As with the 'cold', dementia is a group name for symptoms that may accompany these diseases or conditions.

Some facts and figures (sources: Alzheimer's Society, UK and Alzheimer's Association, USA):

- Now (2018) there are 850,000 people with dementia in the UK.

- There will be one million people with dementia in the UK by 2025. This will soar to two million by 2051.

- Now (2018) there are 5.5 million people with dementia in the USA.

- There could be 16 million people with dementia in the USA by 2050.

- The proportion of people with dementia doubles for every five-year age group.

- One in six people aged 80 and over have dementia.

- Dementia is the leading cause of all deaths in England and Wales (12% in 2017).

- The financial cost of dementia to the UK is £26.3 billion per annum (2018).

- The financial cost of dementia to the USA is $259 billion per annum (2018).

Not everyone who has dementia will experience the same symptoms – indeed there is a saying in the field that 'when you have met a person with dementia, you have met one person with dementia'.

I like to use a physical example to illustrate how the experience of dementia is not the same for everyone. Physical disability can have many causes and will affect people differently depending on what the cause is, where the injury is and what the injured site does.

Take a knee injury, for example; there can be many causes of this:

- arthritis

- damaged bone (perhaps from a fall)

- damaged cartilage (perhaps from overuse, such as jogging)

- damaged ligament (perhaps from twisting during playing football or skiing).

Whatever the cause, the resulting damage impairs the function of the knee. As you know, the knee has several functions and the injury will therefore affect more than one function:

- The knee is a joint that allows the leg to be flexible, so there will be less flexibility for movement and balance.

- The knee is a shock absorber, so any movement on uneven or hard ground will be restricted.

- The knee allows the leg to be stable and supports the person's balance when standing still, so there is more risk of falling.

In addition, an injured knee will be painful, so the person with a knee injury is less likely to want to move or bear weight on it. Impairment of the knee function can disable a person, restricting or stopping their ability to drive, walk, go up and down steps or get in and out of the bath.

As I have said, there are many neurological conditions (diseases of the nerves and brain cells) that can cause dementia. The most common causes are Alzheimer's disease, vascular disease and Lewy body disease. These conditions damage different parts of the brain and cause those parts to not work so well. Of course, the brain is highly complex; with on average

86 billion neurons and 86 trillion connections, it has many more functions than the knee.

Some of those brain functions (known as cognitive processes) help us to engage with other people, and other brain functions help us to engage with objects and with our surroundings and to use reasoning, planning and judgement in order to carry out activities.

I am not going to describe the neurological conditions here. There are many books and websites where that information can be easily obtained. However, you may have noticed that I have referred to 'disability' and I do want to explore more the widely held view of the symptoms of dementia as a disability (difficulty in doing things) caused by the impairments of brain function combined with other circumstances. This is important because, if you agree with this viewpoint, you will immediately be able to see how we can seek to overcome or reverse this disability through rehabilitation approaches.

In order to support understanding of the complex experience of living with dementia, Tom Kitwood described the many factors we must take into account. He proposed a holistic, person-centred approach that considers the personality, life history, health, neurological status and the social-emotional experience of the individual as essential to understanding their unique experience of the condition.

Tom and his colleague, Kathy Bredin, used this formula in order to aid understanding of the unique experience of every individual with dementia (**D**):

$$D = P + B + H + NI + SP$$

Personality: the unique characteristics of individuals will affect their ways of dealing with situations and events. Personality type will affect how a person deals with loss and change and will add to or reduce the signs and symptoms of dementia.

Think of personality traits: introvert, extrovert, adapt, cope, ignore, deny, cover up, give up – each of these will cause the person to act in a different way in response to their own insight into their changing cognitive abilities and also in response to the way that others begin to behave towards them when the signs and symptoms of the brain cell damage become evident.

Biography: life history shapes personality and how we have learned to respond to situations. So past experiences affect all our current behaviour and responses, regardless of any brain cell damage. Combine that with present damaged cognitive abilities, for example, to reason, remember, make judgements, and the person's previously learned patterns of behaviour will be the default response to present situations without doing the thinking but simply acting on the feeling.

Health: physical and mental health affect how we behave. Behaviour can be mistaken by others for signs of 'dementia' when it may be a sign of ill health – for example, someone pacing because they are in pain or becoming isolated because of depression. I will give an example of how this kind of mistake can lead to all sorts of problems when we look at what may be mistaken for dementia later.

Neurological Impairment: cognitive limitations related to damage to nerve cells in the brain. These limitations impair the function that is governed by the damaged area.

Social Psychology: this is the way that the attitudes of others and interactions with others affect the emotional state of a person and can either enhance or limit opportunities to be a part of their social group and to engage in social and individual activity.

So, as you will appreciate, this formula has moved us a long way from the previously dominant biomedical focuses on brain cell damage being the only cause of dementia. That formula would have simply read D = NI and relied on a cure for the brain cell damage. Hence the major pharmaceutical companies' involvement in research and development of anti-dementia drugs. Having said that, however, the drugs we do have currently address the chemical imbalances in the brain rather than the disease process or the resulting damage leading to those imbalances.

D = NI, or How our brain chemicals work and what the drugs do

Every time you move a muscle and every time you think a thought, your nerve cells are hard at work. They are processing information: receiving signals, deciding what to do with them, and dispatching new messages off to their neighbours. Some nerve cells communicate directly with muscle cells, sending them the signal to contract or expand. Other nerve cells are involved solely in communicating with each other. This processing of information must be fast in order to keep up with the ever-changing demands of life and the speed of these messages travelling in the brain can be up to 268 miles per hour.

Brain chemicals

Nerves communicate with one another and with muscle cells by using chemicals known as neurotransmitters. These are small molecules that are released from the nerve cell and rapidly pass to neighbouring cells, stimulating a response once they arrive. Many different neurotransmitters are used for different jobs: glutamate excites nerves into action; GABA inhibits the passing of information; dopamine and serotonin are involved in the subtle messages of thought and cognition. The main job of the neurotransmitter acetylcholine is to carry the signal from nerve cells to muscle cells. It also has a significant role in memory function and the promotion of REM sleep, and it has recently been suggested that acetylcholine disruption may be a primary cause of depression.

Once a chemical message has passed from one cell to the next, the neurotransmitter must be destroyed, otherwise later signals would get mixed up in a jumble of obsolete neurotransmitter molecules. The clean-up of old acetylcholine is the job of acetylcholinesterase (pronounced ass-ee-tile-coal-in-est-er-ayze).

Acetylcholinesterase is found in the synapse between nerve cells and muscle cells. It waits patiently and springs into action soon after a signal is passed, breaking down the acetylcholine into its two component parts, acetic acid and choline. This effectively stops the signal, allowing the pieces to be recycled and rebuilt into new neurotransmitters for the next message. Acetylcholinesterase has one of the fastest reaction rates of any of our enzymes, breaking up each molecule in about 80 microseconds.

Anti-dementia drugs mainly focus on removing or blocking acetylcholinesterase in an attempt to reverse the symptoms of Alzheimer's disease. The progress of the Alzheimer's disease however, does not stop. The pathology of brain cell damage continues and people with Alzheimer's disease lose many nerve cells as the disease progresses. By taking a drug that partially blocks acetylcholinesterase, the levels of the neurotransmitter acetylcholine can be raised, strengthening the nerve signals that remain.

The medication doesn't work for everyone and for some there are horrible side effects of nausea, diarrhoea and vomiting. If an individual comes off the medication, the progression of the Alzheimer's disease is plain as the symptoms of dementia become significantly worse.

So what if there were a more natural way of addressing those chemical imbalances and enabling our brain cells to connect with each other? I would like you to hold onto that thought while we explore more of the approach to understanding dementia by going beyond the brain cell damage from the neurological condition.

D = H + NI, or What may be mistaken for dementia

Now we are going to take a look at more of Tom Kitwood's factors and how they can combine to form the symptoms of dementia. 'H' stands for health and there are some physical and mental health conditions which can be mistaken for dementia. Not only that, they are more likely to be experienced by someone who already has dementia, making the symptoms of dementia worse. And even more worrying, having these health conditions put individuals more at risk of developing dementia than if they didn't have the health condition.

Understanding and treating or preventing these health problems is therefore vital.

Delirium is a sudden and severe change in brain function that causes a person to be confused, disoriented, or to have difficulties maintaining focus, thinking clearly and remembering recent events. Delirium can be triggered by a serious medical illness such as an infection, certain medications and other causes, such as drug withdrawal or intoxication. Older people, over 65 years, are at the highest risk for developing delirium.

People with dementia are particularly vulnerable to delirium because their thinking, reasoning and other cognitive skills can lead to poor diet, not drinking enough liquids, taking too many medications or at the wrong time or in the wrong way, not having good oral hygiene and not controlling the home environment safely – with a risk of carbon monoxide poisoning, for example.

For people who already have the symptoms of dementia, or for older people in general where the ill-informed assume that confusion must be dementia, the risk of it not being recognised and addressed is a major issue.

This is significant when you realise that having a delirium increases the risk of developing dementia eightfold in older patients. Dr Daniel Davis, lead author of a paper from the University of Cambridge, said: 'This means that delirium, or the acute causes of delirium, could be a newly discovered cause of dementia. This is important, because although delirium is extremely common, less than a quarter of cases are actually diagnosed' (2012).

What causes delirium?

The function of the body is a delicate balance of chemistry and physics and, as we age, this can become more difficult to sustain. A high body temperature that can occur as a natural response to fight infections can lead to an imbalance which can, in turn, lead to delirium.

Carbon monoxide poisoning from faulty gas appliances or from burning domestic fuels such as gas, coal, wood and charcoal in an enclosed room, or medication poisoning from taking the wrong dosage or taking medications that interact badly with each other can also lead to delirium.

But toxic states also result from being dehydrated or from not getting the right nutrients, vitamins and minerals. It can be clearly seen that a healthy diet and a full intake of vitamins and minerals will help to prevent health problems causing or adding to dementia. I will be looking at this in great detail and offering you a strategy for maintaining the body balance in Chapter 4.

For those people who need more help in actually getting the food and drink they need into their body we will also be offering you a strategy for addressing cognitive impairments that may stand in their way in Chapter 6.

D = H + NI + SP, or How others can cause dementia

Finally, in this chapter we are going to look at how the symptoms of dementia can be caused or added to by the beliefs, attitudes and approaches of others.

The best way of illustrating this is by telling you this true story of an incident that happened to a patient of mine.

Joan had been in hospital following a fall. It had been assessed that she was unsafe to use the stairs and that she needed a stairlift. However, because she had dementia, it was not clear if she would be able to learn to use the stairlift. So, Joan was referred to me for a cognitive assessment to determine her learning ability.

When I arrived at her cottage, Joan was making a hot drink for her and her husband. They greeted me warmly and Joan agreed to my carrying out some cognitive assessments with her. As these progressed, it became clear to me that Joan did not have any cognitive difficulties and her husband was becoming aware too that her answers to my questions were all correct. He must have been worried that I would not arrive at the 'correct' conclusion so, as his wife turned away, he made a gesture: pointing to his own temple and making a small circular motion to indicate madness. At that same moment, Joan turned back and saw this terrible comment on her mental status. Of course, she was very angry. Her eyes filled with tears and she shouted at him and banged the table with her fist. Her husband rolled his eyes and said: 'See what I mean?' He saw her behaviour as aggression relating to her dementia and her refusal to accept her diagnosis as a lack of insight caused by her dementia.

If Joan had not had the diagnosis, I am certain that her very natural response to the undermining behaviour of her husband would have been viewed very differently. He would have been blamed for his insensitive action, not her for her response to it. And I was not at all convinced that Joan did have dementia.

I was interested to learn more about how her diagnosis had been arrived at. It quickly unfolded that while in hospital Joan had experienced a urinary tract infection which had caused her to be confused, muddled in her thinking and in her speech. In other words, she had a delirium, not dementia and when her infection was treated with antibiotics, the confusion went away. Unfortunately, someone had already attached the label of 'dementia' to her behaviour (perhaps making an assumption based on her age) and this was what she had to fight against. Every time she tried to do so, it was seen as further proof of the condition that she actually didn't have.

You will be pleased to know that the diagnosis was removed and Joan did indeed learn to use her stairlift.

Imagine how much worse this could have been, although that at first doesn't seem possible, if Joan had already had a neurological condition that was causing dementia. It is likely that her increase in confusion would have been attributed to her 'dementia getting worse' and that her infection may not have been investigated or treated.

Joan's experience is unfortunately not an isolated incident but all too real an example of what happens when assumptions that are based on myths and stereotypes are made.

You could actually add the final two factors from Tom Kitwood's equation into Joan's story, because her personality and life story probably caused her to react as she did to each of the injustices that she was experiencing. Our social responses and emotional behaviour are a combination of learning from experience and of personality type. She was a fighter. Imagine if she had not been: would she have given up under the weight of expectation on her to act as if she had dementia? Would that have become a self-fulfilling prophecy?

Whilst of course we cannot alter past life history or personality, we can certainly affect all of the other factors in that equation: health, neurological impairment and social psychology. This is the case for rementia.

Chapter 3

The Case for Rementia

The older view was that there can only be a one-way journey, from the left to the right. Now, however, as a richer body of evidence becomes available…that view is no longer tenable. Some people undergo a degree of 'rementing'.

Tom Kitwood (1997), *Dementia
Reconsidered: The Person Comes First*

Rementia, broken into syllables, is a 'return to the mind.' Better yet, rementia is a 'return to the wellness of the mind'.

Kassandra King (2014), *Getting REAL About Alzheimer's:
Rementia through Engagement, Assistance, and Love*

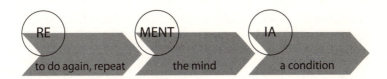

As far back as the late 1980s a school of thought was emerging that challenged the belief that dementia was an irreversible condition. Andrew Sixsmith's paper argued against the 'bio-medical' model of dementia where neurological changes in the brain are believed to lead to an inevitable and progressive decline in the individual's cognitive powers and functional ability (1993). His suggestion was that the social and care context within which the person lives can have a considerable impact on the progress of dementia with the possibility of some degree of 'rementia', the regaining of lost cognitive and functional abilities, when a more positive approach to dementia care is well supported.

This view builds on the idea that society as a whole and individuals within that society can either enable or disable others by their attitudes and approaches. We will be exploring this more in Chapter 5.

On top of addressing the social psychology of dementia though, we now have two other important factors to work with: health and, in particular, nutrition and cognition or neurological impairment.

A person-centred, holistic approach is at the heart of rementia. Wonderfully, this approach gives us more than one opportunity for following a system that achieves improvement in cognitive ability and function. It is possible to address health, emotions and cognition in order to restore function so that an individual no longer has the symptoms of dementia, has fewer symptoms or has less disabling or distressing symptoms.

In his 2014 paper on the reversal of cognitive decline by using a therapeutic system of several approaches Dale Bredesen argues that neurodegenerative disease therapeutics has been till now, arguably, the field of greatest failure. He says that patients with acute illnesses, such as infectious diseases, or with other chronic conditions, such as cardiovascular disease and cancer, have access to more effective therapeutic options than do patients with Alzheimer's disease or other neurodegenerative diseases. Therapeutic success for other chronic illnesses has been improved through the use of combination therapies. Now the past few decades of genetic and biochemical research have revealed an extensive network of molecular interactions involved in Alzheimer's disease that suggest that a network-based therapeutics approach may be feasible and more effective for the treatment of cognitive decline due to Alzheimer's disease. Bredesen presents a system that includes nutrition, stress reduction, sleep optimisation, exercise and brain stimulation. With all of these, apart from brain stimulation, he gives precise guidance for implementing the approach.

My experience is that we can also be focused in not only stimulating the brain but in stimulating cognitive activity in order to reduce the disability of dementia.

The concept of dementia as a disability is now firmly recognised. The UK Government has issued guidelines on disability rights (2015). It states that a mental health condition is considered a disability if it has a long-term effect on normal day-to-day activity. The condition is 'long term' if it lasts, or is likely to last, 12 months. And dementia is explicitly included as one of the conditions. 'Normal day-to-day activity' is defined as something you do regularly in a normal day, for example getting washed and dressed, eating a meal, using a computer or interacting with people.

So, apart from the financial and legal opportunities that this disability status confers, it also follows that where there is disability, there is also potential for rehabilitation.

As Tom Kitwood (1997) said, if we lose faith in people with brain conditions, the chances of rementia are slim. But I would like to add that with belief, will, knowledge and skills the chances of rementia are enormous.

The idea of rementia signifies a phenomenon that is crucial for accepting the idea of recovery without drugs. And yet, this idea is well known to caregivers. There are reports in detailed case studies of individuals with Alzheimer's disease who had, apparently, gone far down the path of behavioural and cognitive impairment, then regained some of their lost abilities. Sometimes this has been in response to the support of particular persons and in some cases it has been evoked by the opportunity to carry out long-practised and highly familiar activities.

You may be questioning how it is possible for a damaged brain to repair itself.

It was once believed that as we aged, the brain's networks became fixed. In the past two decades, however, an enormous amount of research has revealed that the brain never stops changing and adjusting.

You may have heard that the brain is plastic. This refers to the brain's ability to change, reorganising itself by forming new connections between brain cells (neurons) in response to new experiences.

In addition to genetic factors, the environment in which a person lives, as well as the actions of that person, play a role in plasticity which can occur at the beginning of life, when the immature brain organises itself; throughout adulthood, when-ever something new is learned and memorised; and, in the case of brain injury, to compensate for lost functions or maximise remaining functions.

A surprising consequence of neuroplasticity is that the brain activity associated with a given function can move to a different location as a consequence of normal experience, brain damage or recovery.

In his book, *The Brain That Changes Itself: Stories of Personal Triumph from the Frontiers of Brain Science* (2007), Norman Doidge describes numerous examples of functional shifts. In one of them, a surgeon in his 50s had a stroke. His left arm was paralysed. During his rehabilitation, his unaffected arm and hand were immobilised, and he was set to cleaning tables. The task at first was impossible. Then slowly the affected arm remembered how to move. He learned to write again, to play tennis again: the functions of the brain areas killed in the stroke had transferred themselves to healthy regions!

The brain compensates for damage by reorganising and forming new connections between intact neurons. In order to reconnect, the neurons need to be stimulated through activity. You can listen to Dr Doidge speaking about this phenomenon called brain plasticity in an interview by following the link in the References and Reading List (Doidge n.d.).

Recent scientific papers are not questioning the idea of reversing the symptoms of dementia by using rehabilitation approaches. This is now established as an evidence-based practice. Papers such as those published by Macoir and colleagues (2014) and Giebel and Challis (2015) are now more concerned with developing proven interventions in order to achieve this rehabilitation.

My own work has been to develop these interventions and in Chapter 6 I will describe what cognition is, how cognitive impairment disables us and how it is possible to apply interventions that stimulate the activity that is needed to restore cognitive abilities and therefore improve function.

Chapter 4

Cognitive Rehabilitation
Nutrition, or How What You Put in Your Body Affects Your Brain

Nutrition is the process by which we obtain and use food for our body functions. We are guided by research and by politicians as to what foods give us the nutrients that we need. And we are influenced by food sellers and the media as to what foods we consume.

National dietary guidelines were introduced in 1977 and 1983, by the US and UK Governments respectively, with the ambition of reducing coronary heart disease (CHD) by reducing fat intake. However, in 2015, Zoe Harcombe published compelling evidence in the *British Medical Journal* that these dietary recommendations were introduced for 220 million US and 56 million UK citizens in the absence of any supporting evidence from randomised controlled trials.

Her work as an obesity researcher and nutritional therapist challenges the current dietary advice. She defends foods that we have been advised are bad for us (red meat and fats) and exposes non-evidence-based nutritional messages (e.g., 'five a day', the calorie theory, 'healthy' whole-grains, why we can't eat less sugar and more carbs). Zoe also loathes and exposes conflicts of interest – rarely more lucrative or prevalent than where drug or food companies are involved.

Because I do not have the same level of understanding about diet and nutrition as Zoe and other researchers, I am referring you to their work. I have also drawn on the work of Sophie Murray, a nutritional therapist and Head of Nutrition and Hydration with Sunrise Senior Living. Later in this chapter we will be looking at addressing malnutrition, including the use of supplements. There is much evidence that there is a nutrition gap which makes a favourable (some would say essential) case for supplementation. If you do decide to add supplements to your diet, you will need to buy them from a reputable source. Please do first have a complete medical check-up and only take supplements with the guidance of your nutritional therapist.

In trying to understand why obesity increased almost tenfold in the UK between 1972 and 1999 Zoe looked for what had changed. She found that our dietary advice was the thing that changed. We demonised fat; we praised carbohydrate – and epidemics of obesity and type 2 diabetes occurred.

Grain Brain by Dr David Perlmutter (2014), a neurologist in the USA, explains very clearly and with numerous examples how modern wheat, gluten and a diet rich in carbohydrates and sugars cause inflammation in the brain. His book is mainly about Alzheimer's disease and the action you can take to alter your nutritional intake through diet in order to prevent it, but he also includes other neurological conditions such as Parkinson's disease and multiple sclerosis.

Dale Bredesen describes how cognitive decline can be reversed by using a comprehensive and personalised therapeutic programme that is based on the underlying development of Alzheimer's disease. It involves multiple approaches designed to achieve metabolic enhancement to address and reverse neurological conditions. These are primarily diet to minimise inflammation with low glycemic, low grain diets.

All of these authors, and many more that they reference in their works, identify the probable causes of brain cell deterioration (beyond what is expected for normal ageing) as linked to a combination of factors:

- genetics

- lifestyle

- environment.

Genetics

A common question I get asked is: 'My Mum had dementia, so will I get it?' and people are naturally concerned that they may pass it on to their own children.

Alzheimer's disease is the most common cause of dementia and the one that is most understood with regards to genetics. The disease has two main forms: the rare early onset Alzheimer's disease, where symptoms begin before the age of 65; and the more common late onset Alzheimer's disease where symptoms develop later in life. Each of these types has a different pattern of genetic inheritance which increases the risk of developing the disease but neither will lead to a definite development of the disease.

If you are worried about inheriting a condition that causes the symptoms of dementia you should speak to your doctor. Genetic testing is not a straightforward issue and individuals need to think very carefully before deciding to take such a test. The experience might be very difficult emotionally, may not provide conclusive results either way, and may cause practical difficulties.

On the positive side, genetic testing might help genetic researchers understand the conditions better and so lead to improved treatment, encourage someone to adopt a healthier lifestyle or help people to plan for the future.

Although genes are important in building our bodies, most of our physical characteristics and the diseases we may experience are also greatly influenced by our environment and lifestyle, which act to modify the effects of our genetic inheritance.

Environment and lifestyle

Age is the most significant known risk factor for developing the symptoms of dementia, with the risk doubling every five years after the age of 65. It is estimated that one in 14 people over the age of 65 is affected and that this increases to one in six over the age of 80. However, it is helpful to reverse these figures in order to realise that the majority of older people do not have dementia.

So, dementia is not an inevitable part of ageing and it is likely that a combination of environmental and lifestyle factors, plus a genetic predisposition, is the cause.

Here is the list of these main lifestyle factors, which I will describe in a little more detail:

- environmental toxins

- inflammation

- gluten

- cholesterol

- oxidative stress

- high blood sugars.

Environmental toxins

You will most likely have read about the potential impact of chemicals on our body systems and there are many well researched, scientifically robust studies mixed up alongside some questionable media stories. The chemicals range from those in our food chain such as fertilisers, fungicides, pesticides and growth factors such as hormones and antibiotics to chemicals added to foods during processing for enhancing colour or flavour or to preserve, emulsify, glaze or set a food product. In addition, toxins are everywhere from, for example, traffic fumes, cleaning chemicals and beauty products.

It may be difficult to avoid all of the potential toxins, but you may decide to try to avoid some of them. The Alzheimer's Society web page, 'Science behind the headlines' (2015), is a good starting point to get more information on each of these topics. It will help you to see where the consensus lies from considering a range of studies. This is not to be taken as advice but simply an examination of the science behind current claims and studies that are reported in the press. It will be a useful page to keep updated as new stories break.

Inflammation

I think that we all are familiar with inflammation as a healing process by our immune system that involves pain, redness and swelling in response to an injury. But did you know that there is evidence of a strong relationship between inflammation within the brain and dementia? There is also emerging new evidence that the inflammatory responses in other parts of the body may cross the 'blood–brain barrier' and also lead to damage to brain function (Ellison 2017; Heneka *et al.* 2015; Perry *et al.* 1997).

While inflammation is part of the body's natural healing process, excessive inflammation is considered to be one of the leading drivers of the most serious diseases that we are dealing with today. These diseases include diabetes, arthritis, heart disease, Alzheimer's, Parkinson's and many types of cancer. So, what is causing the excessive inflammation in our brains?

A major theory is that the shift in our diets away from natural foods such as wild lean meat, fish, green leafy vegetables, fruit, nuts, berries and honey towards cereal grains as our staple food is the cause (Perlmutter 2014; Vauzoura *et al.* 2017). Added to that is the move away from a diet that was equally balanced between omega-3 and omega-6 essential fatty acids (EFAs).

We have seen a steady increase in our food of omega-6 EFAs at the expense of omega-3 EFAs. Omega-6 fatty acids are cheap and found in all sorts of processed foods and in many vegetable oils. The problem is that omega-6 fatty acids are pro-inflammatory whereas omega-3 is anti-inflammatory.

Gluten

Adding to the effect of the wrong fatty acids, we have also seen a rise in the last 50 years or so of chronic systemic inflammation caused by the increasing use of gluten in our food. In *Grain Brain* (2014), Dr Perlmutter says: 'Gluten is not a single molecule, but two main groups of proteins, glutenins and gliadins, either of which could cause sensitivity reaction (inflammation)' (p.50).

Gluten is a general name for the proteins found in wheat, rye and barley. It helps foods maintain their shape, acting as a glue that holds food together. Gluten can be found in many types of foods, even in some that you would not expect. Apart from the obvious bread, cakes, pasta and biscuits, it is also widely used in processed foods including soups, ice-creams and condiments.

The two main proteins in gluten, glutenin and gliadin, improve both the strength and stickiness of dough. Because of this ability, gluten is a favoured ingredient in the food industry. It helps trap and hold air bubbles during the rising stage so baked products use gluten to help the dough rise and expand.

Bakers often add extra amounts of wheat gluten to recipes that require volume and expansion, such as bread loaves and dinner rolls.

So, gluten is mainly used for volume. Not only does this mean that bread is softer and more appealing to the consumer, it also enables food companies to decrease costs while increasing the size of a product. It could be argued that companies are responding to consumer demand for soft bread or that companies have been adding gluten to get a better return on their products. It is probably a combination of both factors, pleasure and profit, but, either way, possibly at the expense of our health.

There is increasing awareness of the problems that gluten causes to our digestive system and many people are aware of gluten sensitivity that leaves them feeling bloated and in discomfort or pain. This same sensitivity also affects the brain, leading to inflammation. In fact, the brain cells are more prone to damage from gluten than the digestive system.

The body's inflammatory response to gluten produces cytokines which travel around the body and, when they cross the blood–brain barrier, they block the production of chemicals called neurotransmitters. These chemicals are needed for carrying messages from one brain cell to another. In addition, cytokines bind to the brain cells and cause inflammation. This inflammation leads to the production of more cytokines in the brain and a vicious cycle has begun.

Professor Marios Hadjivassilou at Sheffield's Royal Hallamshire Hospital is one of the most respected researchers of gluten sensitivity and the brain. In his studies, he concludes that gluten sensitivity is common in patients with neurological disease. Evidence points to the nervous system as the prime site of gluten damage (1996, 2002).

On top of all this damage, vitamin and mineral deficiencies are linked to a high gluten diet. I will be explaining more about vitamins and minerals in a moment. But, it is alarming to realise that gluten 'hijacks' these essential nutrients so they can then not be absorbed by the body.

Cholesterol

The brain thrives on a fat-rich, low-carbohydrate diet. As this goes against the current dietary advice this type of diet is relatively uncommon in human populations today. Dr Perlmutter explains in *Grain Brain* (2014) that carbohydrates typically thought of as healthy (such as brown rice, 100% whole-grain bread, or quinoa) cause disorders like dementia over a lifetime of consumption. These carbohydrates are now thought by many to be the true source of problems that plague our brains and hearts. By removing these inflammation-causing carbohydrates from the diet and increasing the amount of fat and cholesterol we consume, we can not only protect our most valuable organ, but also potentially undo years of damage. Cholesterol, for example, long vilified by the media and medical community, actually *promotes* neurogenesis (the birth of new brain cells) and communication between neurons, to the degree that studies have shown that higher levels of serum cholesterol correlate to more robust cognitive prowess.

Zoe Harcombe, a leading nutritional therapist, believes that we have got cholesterol completely wrong. She says that it is virtually impossible to explain how vital cholesterol is to the human body:

> If you had no cholesterol in your body you would be dead. No cells, no bone structure, no muscles, no hormones, no sex, no reproductive system, no digestion, no brain function, no memory, no nerve endings, no movement, no human life – nothing without cholesterol. It is utterly vital and we die instantly without it. (Harcombe n.d.)

Harcombe explains that cholesterol is so vital to the body that our bodies make it themselves. The body cannot risk leaving it to chance that we would get it externally from food or some other external factor – that's how critical it is.

There is increasing evidence that most modern diseases are brought about by chronic inflammation, not the kind that occurs when you're injured and the injury site begins to swell, but the kind that is wreaking havoc at the cellular level in the bodies of most people every day. Low immune response due to lack of nutritional support does not allow the body to protect and heal itself. Despite previous medical and pharmaceutical consensus, new studies are showing that dietary cholesterol may actually *stop* inflammation, prevent blood clots from forming, support the immune system, and prevent disease causing mutations in cells.

Harcombe explains that there is no such thing as good cholesterol and bad cholesterol. Cholesterol is cholesterol. HDL and LDL are not forms of cholesterol. HDL stands for high density lipoprotein. LDL stands for low density lipoprotein. Lipoproteins are *carriers* of cholesterol as well as other substances. LDL would more accurately be called the carrier of fresh cholesterol and HDL would more accurately be called the carrier of recycled cholesterol.

One in 500 people have familial hypercholesterolemia and may have a problem clearing cholesterol in their body (rather like type 1 diabetics who can't return their blood glucose levels to normal). For anyone else to be actively trying to lower their vital and life-affirming cholesterol levels is deeply troubling.

Oxidative stress

Several studies suggest that oxidative stress may play a role in the changes in the brain that cause Alzheimer's disease.

Free radicals are produced by cells as a by-product of energy production, and therefore are a result of normal functioning. In the brain, free radicals seem to contribute to ageing and age-associated neurodegenerative disorders. The brain is particularly susceptible to oxidative damage as it uses lots of oxygen to produce energy, has high levels of unsaturated fatty acids (which are particularly susceptible to damage), and relatively low levels of antioxidants. There is substantial evidence that oxidative damage to the brain is an early event in Alzheimer's disease. Brains of people with Alzheimer's disease appear to have higher levels of natural antioxidants responsible for 'clearing up' excess free radicals, suggesting that the body is trying to combat this damage. Signs of oxidative stress are found not only in the brain, but also in the cerebral spinal fluid and the urine of people with Alzheimer's disease.

To prevent this damage, our bodies naturally make, and acquire from food, molecules that react with free radicals. These are generally called 'antioxidants'.

Huge numbers of different substances can act as anti-oxidants. Some of the most well known include vitamin C, vitamin E, betacarotene and other related carotenoids, flavonoids, phenols, and many more. Putting all these chemicals into one large group is actually quite misleading. Each antioxidant has a different chemical composition, behaves slightly differently and has a slightly different role. However, a diet rich in antioxidants is thought to be helpful in preventing or reducing the symptoms of dementia.

High blood sugars

Brain chemicals are called neurotransmitters and these pass messages from one brain cell to the next, enabling us to function. When blood sugar levels rise, there is an immediate corres-ponding reduction in the levels of several neurotransmitters.

Additionally, high blood sugars trigger a reaction called 'glycation' where sugar molecules and proteins combine to form deadly new structures in the brain that are stiff and inflexible, causing degeneration of the brain and its function. There is increasing evidence of a risk relationship between diabetes and dementia.

In people with diabetes, higher levels of glucose in cells leads to glycation – the increase in the uncontrolled production of protein and glucose compounds. Increasing evidence suggests that glycation is a key factor in age-related neurological conditions such as Alzheimer's disease and Parkinson's disease. The link between diabetes and dementia is unclear, but neurological problems do tend to occur more frequently in people with diabetes. While more studies are being carried out, we do not yet have the full picture, but it makes sense to keep blood sugar levels under control for body and brain health.

In summary, there is a set of potential factors that that lead to the symptoms of dementia and we do not yet know if it is one or the other or a combination of these factors. Gluten, sugar and pro-inflammatory foods and toxins appear to be high risk. So, while we wait for the researchers to come up with the answers, perhaps it would be a good idea to address our own lifestyle with a multi-therapeutic approach to nutrition with a diet that:

- is anti-inflammatory

- is low in omega-6 fatty acids and high in omega-3 EFAs

- is gluten-free

- maintains cholesterol

- includes antioxidants

- helps eliminate toxins

- doesn't generate high blood sugars.

Warning: undernutrition and malnutrition alert!

On top of paying some serious attention to what foods we should and should not be eating, you may like to know more about the risks of undereating.

The Alzheimer's Disease International (2014) report, 'Nutrition and dementia', identifies that, in developed countries, 10 per cent of older people living at home, 30 per cent of those living in care homes and 70 per cent of hospitalised older people suffer from undernutrition.

They say that there are many dietary factors that might plausibly increase or decrease risk for the onset of dementia. The fact is that 20–45 per cent of those with dementia in the community experience clinically significant weight loss over one year, and up to half of people with dementia in care homes have an inadequate food intake.

Undernutrition results from an imbalance between nutrient/ energy intake and needs. This is usually due to an inadequate diet, but can also be the result of altered digestion, absorption and metabolism of nutrients and energy from foods.

Fact: Evidence on the association between dementia and weight loss is compelling.

It seems that not getting enough energy into our bodies can be one of the causes of dementia and also that those who have dementia are more likely to be at risk of undernutrition, leading to their symptoms of dementia getting worse.

It follows, therefore, that if we understand why an individual with dementia is experiencing undernutrition, we can support them to get more nutrients and energy and so reverse some of the symptoms or the degree of dementia.

There are many reasons why a person with dementia might be undernourished. My own experiences with Mum and with my many patients help to shed light on why people with dementia are at risk of becoming undernourished because of their cognitive difficulties. For example, one day when I joined Mum for lunch at her care home I noticed that the housekeeper served the meals and then left the dining room. The support staff were busy helping residents who had remained in their own rooms to eat. I was seated at a table with Mum and another lady who clearly had perceptual problems. The food was in front of her and a spoon was in her hand but she was unable to connect the two. The housekeeper returned and gently reminded the lady to eat but, as this wasn't her cognitive problem, the lady continued to simply wave her spoon around. I offered to help her and in response to her grateful acceptance, I guided her spoon-holding hand to the plate by supporting her elbow. The lady needed this level of support every few mouthfuls but in between those she seemed to get into a pattern of eating. She clearly needed someone to sit with her to give this level of support.

Meanwhile, at the next table I noticed that another lady was slumped in front of a plate of sandwiches and appeared not to have noticed them. Her dining partner enthusiastically finished his food and then hers. When the housekeeper returned to clear the empty plates she praised both diners for having such good appetites! That lady needed someone to remind her to eat or maybe she also had perceptual or recognition difficulties.

Both were at risk of undernutrition but an awareness of the risk and an understanding of how to prevent it would save them from a downward spiral into further dementia and other likely health problems.

Further warning: dehydration alert!

Hydration is crucial to good health, impacting on the body's ability to regulate temperature and blood pressure. If you don't drink enough fluids, it increases the risk of urinary tract infections, which can lead to hospital admission in older people. In addition, being dehydrated can decrease your brain function, causing an acute confusional state (sometimes called a delirium).

Dehydration happens when an individual loses more fluids than they take in, which results in the body not having enough fluids to perform normal functions. When mild dehydration occurs, an individual will lose 2 per cent of their body weight. Severe dehydration is when an individual loses at least 4 per cent of their body weight.

The human body, on average, is made up of 55–60 per cent water; however, the water content of a 75- to 80-year-old is nearly 50 per cent less than that of a young person. Without water, the human body is not able to function.

Dehydration is the most common fluid and electrolyte condition in older adults. If left untreated, dehydration can cause serious long-term health effects in older people. And people who are living with dementia are more at risk of dehydration than those without dementia. Here are some of the main reasons why:

- They can forget to drink simply because they forget where they placed their drink or if they even had a drink.

- They cannot recognise when they are thirsty because the area of the brain that will trigger an individual to drink when they are thirsty is affected. In these situations, individuals may feel parched but they are not able to make the connection between taking a drink and relieving their thirst.

- They cannot recognise the cup or mug or the drink in it so even though they recognise their thirst, they cannot satisfy it.

- They cannot initiate the movement to reach out and pick up the cup or mug.

- There are certain medications that are commonly prescribed that can cause a diuretic effect, which will cause frequent urination. This will cause the body to lose fluids quickly. For example, many medications that are used to treat high blood pressure have diuretic effects.

- Certain illnesses can also lead to dehydration, particularly conditions where a person may be vomiting or have diarrhoea.

- The inability to swallow can also lead to dehydration for those with dementia. For some people with dementia, their brain is affected in such a way that the mouth and throat do not receive messages from the brain to tell them what to do when eating or drinking. Or they simply may not like the taste of thickened fluids.

The NHS recommends that we should drink about 1.2 litres (six to eight glasses) of fluid every day to stop us getting dehydrated. In the US, the recommendation is higher, with the general rule of thumb that you should drink eight eight ounce glasses of fluid per day (at least). Juices and sports drinks are also hydrating – you can lower the sugar content by diluting them with water. Coffee and tea also count in your tally. Many used to believe that they were dehydrating, but that myth has been debunked. The diuretic effect does not offset hydration.

In Table 4.1 I have listed the main impairments of brain function that are likely to disable the person in eating and drinking with some examples of how they can be addressed in order to compensate for the difficulties.

In Chapter 6 I will describe how it is possible to apply cognitive approaches that overcome the impairment and restore dining skills.

When we get to the Rementia Plan you will be able to see how these ideas can be brought together as a multi-therapeutic framework for an individual.

Table 4.1. Impairments of brain function and nutrition/hydration

Impairment of brain function and nutrition/ hydration	Disability	Compensatory solution
Appetite or thirst control (e.g. hypothalamus damage)	Not aware when hungry or thirsty or when full	Small regular meals that are timetabled Favourite drinks regularly offered in small cups or mugs
Awareness of time (orientation)	Not aware of the time for eating	Reminders and verbal prompts (real or technology)
Getting started (initiation)	Not able to begin the action to prepare or eat a meal or to reach for a drink	Verbal prompts: reminders and gentle encouragement Visual prompts: shared meal preparation or dining to cue the person to the activity Tactile prompts: placing cutlery or the cup in the person's hands may cue them to start the activity of dining Olfactory prompts: food and drink smells that trigger the process of eating

Recognising objects (perception)	Not able to make links between the use of an object and the eating or drinking activity	Present the information through all of the senses: Vision – familiar objects, strong colours Hearing – music or other medium that is related to the dining time (favourite TV or radio show) Smell – strong, pleasant food aromas Taste – familiar flavours Touch – object contact (cutlery or finger food placed into the hands)
Seeing objects against a background (figure–ground discrimination)	Not able to see cutlery, plates or drinking vessels on the table or food on the plate	Crockery in a strong colour contrast to the tableware Food and drink in a strong colour contrast to the crockery
Movement (sensorimotor actions)	Not responding to the sensation of an object with a corresponding action, e.g. not able to reach out to take food that can be smelled or seen; not able to raise a fork or spoon when it is placed in the hand	Model the action by shared meal preparation or dining and drinking to cue the person to the action Place the object in the person's hand Enable the start of the action by, for example, gently supporting under the elbow and raising the person's arm towards the object or towards the mouth
Doing actions in order (sequencing)	Not able to follow a set of actions from start to finish such as cutting up food–getting food onto a fork–raising fork to the mouth–putting food into the mouth–chewing–swallowing	Break down the activity into smaller stages or into one step at a time

cont.

Impairment of brain function and nutrition/hydration	Disability	Compensatory solution
Slow reasoning	Not able to eat at a pace that enables food to stay appetising or to drink at a pace that enable the drink to stay warm or to fit with the social aspect of dining	Slow the pace of the activity to suit the person Plate small amounts of food and pour small amounts of hot drink and top up when finished with further helpings Serve drinks in insulated vessels
Low concentration level (attention)	Distracted by others and events so not finishing eating or drinking	Minimise distractions – turn off the television, small dining group or lone dining if preferred Plate small amounts of food/serve small drinks and top up when finished with further helpings Offer smaller, more frequent meals and drinks

Poor oral hygiene can add to the problem

In addition, and related to these cognitive impairments, poor oral health is also a risk factor for undernutrition and also for dementia. There is a complex relationship between oral health and brain function. On one level, tooth decay and gum infection cause pain which leads to a reduction in chewing and even to an avoidance of food. The resulting nutritional deficiencies lead to even more cognitive impairment.

A study in 2017 made for sensationalised headlines: 'Gum disease sufferers 70% more likely to get dementia', reported in *The Times* (Smyth 2017). In fact, a more measured analysis of the Taiwanese study can be found at the NHS News online site

(NHS Choices 2017). They explain that the study found that people with a 10-year or longer history of chronic periodontitis (CP) had a small but significant increased risk of developing Alzheimer's disease. The study was felt to raise an important need for further research as it was not possible to tell whether the results were influenced by people having early undiagnosed Alzheimer's disease that may have led to poorer oral hygiene.

Studies by researchers at the University of Central Lancashire (UCLan) School of Medicine and Dentistry in England (Harding *et al.* 2017) suggest that gum disease such as *Porphyromonas gingivalis* infection (gingivitis) can result in the bacteria entering the bloodstream through everyday activities such as eating, chewing and toothbrushing. Once in the bloodstream, the bacteria can be carried to other parts of the body including the brain, where they may trigger an immune system inflammatory response. As we have already seen, an inflammatory immune response could be one mechanism that leads to the changes in the brain, which are typical in Alzheimer's disease.

The answer to studies is simple: pay serious attention to oral hygiene.

Malnutrition

Malnutrition literally means poor or bad nutrition. Researchers are identifying that malnutrition may also contribute to the cause and the effect of dementia. Whilst undernutrition is caused mainly by not eating enough, malnutrition is caused by eating the wrong nutrients or by our body not using the nutrients properly. You will remember that earlier, for example, I outlined how a high gluten diet prevents the absorption of vitamins and minerals and so will lead to malnutrition.

The UK is now recognising the potential benefits of preventing and treating malnutrition and has therefore created a 'Malnutrition Task Force'. Their first report, 'Preventing Malnutrition in Later Life' (Wilson 2013), gives many interesting facts and figures to help our understanding.

Paying attention to a good diet means having the proper balance of nutrients for good health. There are many sources of this information, and I would recommend that you seek out the support of a qualified nutritional therapist.

There are many books and articles in magazines and on the Internet with suggested supplements that may help complement and enhance your nutritional intake. Beware: many of these articles are sensationalised to make a good headline, for example: 'Red wine prevents Alzheimer's'. In fact, as with many of these stories, there is some truth in the claim but it has been distorted. We know, for example, that there seems to be a link between a glass of red wine a day and a healthy heart. And we know that a healthy heart can mean a healthy brain also.

In terms of preventing the symptoms of dementia, we do know that resveratrol has a positive impact on brain cell function – and resveratrol is found in fermented grape skins. Hence the claim for red wine, as white wine is not fermented. But, in order to obtain the required amount of protective resveratrol, you would need to drink 44 glasses of red wine a day. Not to be recommended! So, as with other vitamins, minerals and enzymes, it can be helpful to top up to the optimum levels needed with purchased supplements. These can be in the form of multivitamins that are developed to supply the basic vitamins and supplements that your diet may be lacking. There are also specialised supplements on the market that are aimed specifically at enhancing brain function. However, these have mixed reviews and, before you embark on taking any mineral, vitamin or other supplements, please consult and take advice from a nutritional therapist who will be trained to address any underlying causes, such as the interaction between your medication and your nutrition. A nutritional therapist can help to promote your brain health with a tailored diet and supplement programme. Currently in the UK, GPs are not trained in nutrition, but they can take advice from the nutritional therapist and work in partnership with them and you to maximise your brain health. Dr Rupy Aujla (2017) is a medical doctor specialised in General Practice and is working with the Royal College of General Practitioners GP on the UK's first 'Culinary Medicine' course. The course aims to teach doctors and health professionals the foundations of nutrition. Another pioneer of the 'prescribing lifestyle medication' is Dr Rangan Chatterjee (2017) who promotes the four pillars of diet, exercise, sleep and relaxation for better health and is currently leading courses for GPs on this approach.

Some of the main supplements that you can buy, in multi-products or singly, that are beginning to be recognised as having potential benefits are:

- omega-3 EFA and DHA (docosahexaenoic acid), because they are anti-inflammatory

- resveratrol, because it boosts blood flow to the brain and because it's said to protect cells against a wide range of diseases

- turmeric (curcumin), because it has the ability to activate genes to produce antioxidants that can protect our cells

- probiotics which play a role in creating neurochemicals, such as serotonin and dopamine, which are essential for a healthy brain and nerve function

- alpha lipoic acid, which crosses the blood–brain barrier and acts as an antioxidant in the brain

- vitamin D, because studies have shown that it protects neurons from the damaging effects of free radicals and reduces inflammation

- vitamins C, E, and beta carotene, because they counteract oxidative damage caused by certain foods, such as gluten

- coconut oil, because it's a rich source of ketogenic fats which provide the brain with the energy that it needs and support brain cell repair and recovery.

In summary, this chapter has set out the current thinking about nutrition and how what you put into your body, what you don't put into your body and how much you put into your body affects your brain.

All of these factors are within our own control. The important and exciting message is that we can do something to improve our brain function and to reduce the symptoms of dementia in those who are living with the disability.

I hope that Table 4.1, which highlights for you the range of likely cognitive impairments that someone may experience, is useful too. It should make you think about how you can support the person you know to eat and drink well as one approach to cognitive rehabilitation and rementia.

Chapter 5

Cognitive Rehabilitation

Emotion, or How You What You Feel Affects Your Brain

Fact: Strong emotions make us stupid. (Attributed to Joseph Ledoux, *The Emotional Brain*)

Most of us know that thinking becomes difficult when we are emotionally aroused, for example, angry or frightened. This natural response is a protection in threatening situations, even ensuring our survival when taking action becomes more important than thinking about the situation. Joseph Ledoux (2015) explains how we use our brain to understand and treat fear and anxiety and that anxious people exhibit disrupted cognitive and behavioural control in the presence of threats.

It is useful to understand this process as it will help to make sense of why a person who has the symptoms of dementia may be behaving as they do. That understanding can support you to enable rather than disable the person. In other words, your interaction has the power to reduce the person's disability and move them towards rementia. Or your interaction may undermine the person and make the symptoms of dementia worse.

Our perceptions are processed through the limbic system of the brain before being transferred to the neocortex. The limbic system is a set of primitive brain structures underneath the cortex of the brain. When an emotion is strong, the limbic system will trigger a response before the cortex has had time to become involved. In other words, the response is triggered before we have a chance to think about it.

If the emotion is very strong our brains can and will automatically shut down our rational thinking process and we find ourselves acting entirely on impulse. Strong emotions such as intense fear may immediately put us into a primitive state where our body is set up to either fight or flee for survival. Our thinking may take on an 'all or nothing' or 'black and white' style. We lose the ability to discriminate or to see shades of grey.

Fact: Stress kills brain cells.

The body's stress response is perfect in the short term but damaging if it goes on for weeks or years. Several research programmes have identified a role of stress hormones in the occurrence and progression of cognitive disorders in older people. A major UK Alzheimer's Society funded research project is investigating chronic (long-term) stress as a risk factor for developing dementia.

Lead researcher Clive Holmes (2018) says:

> Understanding the role of the immune system in the risk of Alzheimer's disease is of great importance to researchers. As prolonged stress can cause changes in the immune system, we wanted to find out if this was linked to progression to dementia from mild cognitive impairment.
>
> Our investigations show that stress does appear to have an effect on progression in mild cognitive impairment. Our preliminary (unpublished) findings are showing that this may be mediated through a fault in the regulation of the immune

system in people with mild cognitive impairment but we are continuing to investigate this further.

High levels of stress hormones put the body into a 'catabolic' state. This is the destructive phase of cell life that includes widespread tissue destruction, muscle loss, bone loss, immune system depression and even brain shrinkage.

The stress hormone, cortisol, has been shown to damage and kill cells in the hippocampus (the brain area responsible for the long-term storage and retrieval of memories; Kim, Pellman and Jeansok 2015) and there is robust evidence that chronic stress causes premature brain ageing (Carroll 2002).

The cortisol released in stress travels into the brain and binds to the receptors inside many neurons. Through a cascade of reactions, this causes neurons to admit more calcium through channels in their membrane.

Cortisol is a necessary stress hormone designed to help you wake up in the morning and, in emergencies, to cope with danger. However, if neurons become overloaded with calcium they fire too frequently and die – they are literally excited to death. The idea that chronic stress could lead to dementia risk is worrying, but it is a factor that we have some degree of control over. The findings of current studies have led some researchers to suggest that this knowledge will support the development of anti-stress medication, but my argument is that we can reduce and, even better, prevent chronic stress in more proactive and non-pharmacological therapeutic ways.

Reducing stress through relationship

The person-centred approach was originated by Carl Rogers, an influential American psychologist. This was his unique app-roach to understanding personality and human relationships.

Rogers (1961) described the qualities that contribute to a person-centred environment:

- **Respect** for the experiences of the person, for their rights, their wishes and for their uniqueness of person

- **Non-judgemental acceptance** that does not depend on the abilities, look or actions of the individual

- **Emphasis on feelings** that recognises the quality of the emotional life of the person

- **Holistic approaches** that consider the physical, social, emotional and spiritual needs of each person

- **Emphasis on relationships**, recognising that interactions affect the feelings and the behaviours of others and that relationships do not depend on cognitive skills

- **Positive views** of the nature of humans for growth and development, using an holistic approach that recognises the potential for development in ways that do not rely on cognitive ability

- **Non-directive approach** aiming to support independence and to enhance feelings of self-control.

It is worth exploring the emphasis on relationships as it is the quality of these that leads to the emotions that we feel. Mike Nolan, Professor of Gerontological Nursing, developed the Senses Framework (Nolan *et al.* 2006) for creating an 'enriched environment' where people can experience empowering relationships. He suggests that people need to feel a sense of:

- **security** – to feel safe physically and psychologically

- **belonging** – to feel part of a valued group

- **continuity** – to be able to make links between the past, present and future

- **purpose** – to enjoy meaningful activity

- **achievement** – to reach goals that matter to the person

- **significance** – to feel that you 'matter'.

It is possible to see how these approaches support each other. In an unsupportive relationship, the distress the person feels will affect their ability and can add to their symptoms of dementia. But with a supportive relationship, the ability of the person can improve and the symptoms of dementia can reduce.

So, to go further with the example in the previous chapter on Nutrition, not only can you look at the cognitive impairments that are making it difficult for the person to eat and drink well, but you can also adapt the way you behave with a person as an approach to support their dining experience as an approach to rementia. You could consider these questions when supporting the person to dine well:

Security

- Does the person feel safe on the chair? Is it in the best position for feeling safe, is it stable and firm?

- Does the person feel safe with and trust in the one who is supporting them to eat?

- Does the person feel self-confidence and self-esteem when dining with others?

Belonging

- Does the person feel included in the dining group?

- Are they invited into conversations?
- Do they feel accepted and valued?

Continuity

- Does the person recognise and like the food?
- Does the dining time fit with the person's routines and habits?

Purpose

- Does the person experience the meal as an opportunity to achieve good nutrition, satisfy hunger, enjoy a range of sensory experiences and participate in social relationships?

Achievement

- Does the person manage to use their abilities to enjoy the meal, get the right nutrition and improve or maintain their health and well-being?

Significance

- Did the dining experience make the person feel that they matter?

The principles underpinning these questions can be applied to any activity that the person is engaging in and the questions modified to suit the activity. This then ensures that you are not only considering the steps of the activity but also the social and emotional context of the activity.

Using emotional intelligence

I often ask family and friends who are bewildered and distressed by the conversation and behaviour of a person with dementia to take a step back from trying to work out what the person means and instead focus on what the person is feeling. This is usually a critical moment in developing a supportive relationship for them both.

Emotional intelligence is the ability to identify, use, understand and manage emotions in positive ways to relieve stress, communicate effectively, empathise with others, overcome challenges and defuse conflict.

Emotional intelligence frameworks are used in business and are now being used more in care to support problem solving and effective ways of working with others. Table 5.1 describes Goleman's (1995) four-quadrant model of emotional intelligence which you can use to think about your own feelings and behaviour as well as the feelings and behaviour of others.

Table 5.1. Goleman's (1995) four-quadrant model of emotional intelligence

	Self	Other
Awareness	**Self-awareness** What are you feeling? How did these feelings arise? What do these feelings tell you?	**Social awareness** What are they feeling? How did those feelings arise?
Actions	**Self-management** How do you want to feel? What do you need to do in order to feel that way?	**Relationship management** How do you want them to feel? What do you need to do in order for them to feel that way?

Asking yourself these questions can be a powerful way of changing what you do. By doing so, you can improve the situation for both of you and support the person to be more able in their function and in their communication.

Here is a series of diagrams that I have often used in my teaching programmes for care workers. It illustrates what can go wrong in communication and how that impacts on relationships and on the symptoms of dementia: making them worse or better.

Usually the connection between people is a give-and-take process:

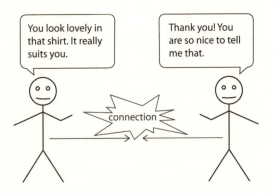

Our 'arrows of connection' are fairly equal.

But, if we don't understand each other, the connection will be missing:

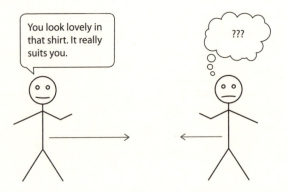

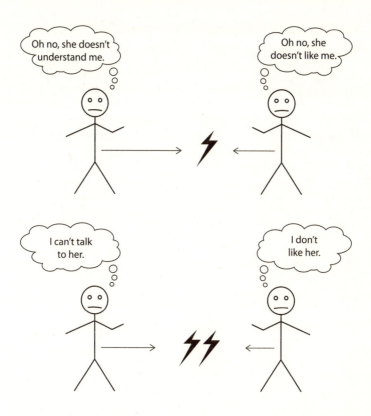

Notice how the ability to connect is reduced for both people (arrows become smaller).

The solution is to first recognise that there is a problem...

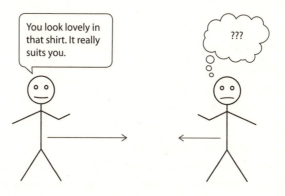

And how that is impacting on the other person…

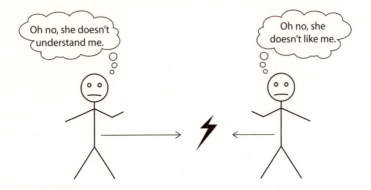

Then, use all your skills and abilities to address the problem…

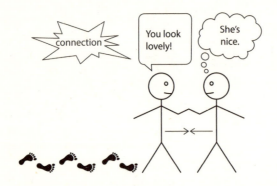

Move your 'arrow of connection' closer to the person by identifying the emotional experience of the person and then nurturing their sense of confidence and self-esteem, by using touch and eye contact and by simplifying your language.

So, how can you use these theoretical approaches to support emotional well-being and achieve a reduction in the symptoms of dementia?

Confidence and self-esteem come from a sense of mattering to others and a feeling of being valued as an individual. We can support that sense or undermine it by the way we are with the person. Table 5.2 has some 'do' and 'don't' Guidelines that will help you to move your arrows of connection closer to each other.

Table 5.2. Social relationships: 'do' and 'don't' guidelines

How can I have a nurturing connection? DO…	How can I avoid an undermining connection? DON'T…
Listen out for tone and volume to understand what content of the conversation is important to the person	Focus only on the facts of the conversation or correct what the person is saying
Look for signs of how the person is feeling and tell them you recognise that (e.g. 'I can see that you are sad')	Ignore their emotional experience or tell them it is not valid (e.g. 'Don't be silly, it's not that bad')
Show a genuine interest in what the person is saying: repeat some of their words, smile and nod	Look bored or confused
Respond to the person's mistaken belief by acknowledging how they are feeling and discussing their subjective experience	Respond to the person's mistaken belief by lying to them or by bluntly correcting them
Have fun with the person	Have fun at the person's expense
Reinforce the person's achievements	Highlight the person's difficulties
Tell the person that you have not understood the meaning of the conversation	Tell the person that they have not been clear in the delivery of their conversation
Give the person information if they are struggling to recall it	Put pressure on the person to remember events, names and other topics of conversation

In addition to nurturing the emotional connection with these few simple guidelines, you can also compensate for the communication disability caused by the cognitive impairments.

In Chapter 4 I showed you how we can address the main impairments of brain function that are likely to disable the person's dining ability. As with the difficulties with eating and drinking, in Table 5.3 I have listed the main impairments of brain function that are likely to disable the person in their communication.

In Chapter 6 I will describe how it is possible to apply cognitive approaches that go beyond compensatory strategies to overcome the impairment and restore communication skills.

When we get to the Rementia Plan you will be able to see how these ideas can be brought together as a multi-therapeutic framework for an individual.

Table 5.3. Impairment of brain function and communication

Impairment of brain function and communication	Disability	Compensatory solution
Understanding spoken language (receptive dysphasia)	Not able to make sense of what is being said	Use gestures, facial expression and tone of voice to add meaning to words Use pictures and objects to illustrate meaning Make sure that the person can see your mouth Enunciate clearly Keep sentences short Cut out unnecessary words
Producing spoken language (expressive dysphasia)	Difficulty finding the right words	Listen for meaning in the person's use of tone Watch for meaning in the person's use of gestures and facial expression Allow time for the person to search for the word If you can understand the meaning, don't correct the person's word use If you can't understand the meaning, ask the person 'Do you mean…?' Learn the person's language – if they have a certain word that they use for a certain meaning

Getting started (initiation)	Not able to begin a conversation	Make the first move – offer topics that you know will interest the person Make eye contact with the person, if possible, before starting to speak
Short-term memory difficulty	Not able to hold onto the topic whilst discussing it Repeating topics of conversation	Regularly refer by name to the topic rather than using a pronoun (he, she, they, it) Subtly remind the person (e.g. 'When we were talking about the weather just now, you said…') Act each time as though it is the first time you have heard it. Pick up on a different element of the topic to continue and move forwards with the conversation
Slow reasoning	Not able to follow the conversation Not able to follow changes of topic	Slow the pace of the conversation to match the person's rate of speech Cue the person to changes of topic (e.g. 'Let's leave that now and talk about this')
Low concentration level (attention)	Distracted by others and events so not able to attend to the conversation	Minimise distractions. For example, turn off the television, reduce noise, hold conversations in a quiet and visually still area Have small social groups Only one person speak at a time
Abstract thinking	Not able to discuss ideas and events that are not 'here and now'	Focus conversation on physical topics rather than on ideas and relationships between those ideas Avoid metaphors and figures of speech unless they are familiar to the person (e.g. 'Let's stretch our legs') Use objects to support the link between a concrete 'here and now' topic and an abstract 'in the past' or 'in the future' topic (e.g. a calendar or a diagram)

I hope that you will see how you can adapt these possible compensatory solutions to other aspects of the person's experience. By doing so, you will reduce their disability of dementia and support their process of rementia. Oh yes, and you will equally benefit with a sense of fulfilment and well-being as your own 'arrow of connection' is being met too!

You might be wondering where these social connections should take place. The place is not so important as the opportunity and the quality of the interaction. The recent WHELD study led by Professor Clive Ballard and Dr Anne Corbett of the University of Exeter (Ballard *et al.* 2018) describes how just one hour a week of social interaction, talking about their lives and interests, can improve well-being and health of people who are living with dementia. These conversations can take place in the person's own home or at social gatherings outside of the home.

A few words about sleep, relaxation and meditation
Sleep deeper and longer
Sleep ranks with diet and regular exercise as an essential component of a healthy life.

The function of sleep has mystified scientists for thousands of years, but modern research is providing new clues about what it does for both the mind and body. Sleep serves to reenergise the body's cells, clear waste from the brain, and support learning and memory. It even plays a vital role in regulating mood, appetite and libido.

Sleeping is an integral part of our life, and as research shows, it is incredibly complex. The brain generates two distinct types of sleep – slow-wave sleep (SWS), known as deep sleep, and rapid eye movement (REM), also called dreaming sleep. Most of the sleeping we do is of the SWS variety, characterised by large, slow brain waves, relaxed muscles and slow, deep breathing, which may help the brain and body to recuperate after a long day.

Deep sleep is one of the most fundamental ways our body heals itself. Without sleep you can't form or maintain the pathways in your brain that let you learn and create new memories, and it is harder to concentrate and respond quickly.

The National Institute of Neurological Diseases and Stroke (NINDS 2017) states that sleep is important to a number of brain functions, including how nerve cells (neurons) communicate with each other. In fact, your brain and body stay remarkably active while you sleep. Recent findings suggest that sleep plays a housekeeping role by removing toxins in your brain that build up while you are awake.

Ideally while you sleep your body should be busy repairing itself, so I'd like to offer you some insight that I think will help you or the person you support to obtain much-needed sleep without the negative side effects of drugs or even supplements like melatonin.

The hormone cortisol can play a major role in robbing someone of a good night's sleep. As discussed earlier in this chapter, cortisol is the necessary 'stress hormone' that is designed to help you wake up in the morning and in emergencies, to cope with danger. However, too much cortisol is a problem and the average 50-year-old has nighttime cortisol levels more than 30 times higher than those of the average 30-year-old.

Circulating cortisol normally rises and falls throughout the 24-hour daily cycle, and is typically highest at around 8 am and lowest between midnight and 4 am.

Stress normally causes a surge in adrenal hormones like adrenaline and cortisol that increase alertness, making it more difficult to relax into sound sleep. Frequent or constant stress can chronically elevate these hormone levels, resulting in a hypervigilant state incompatible with restful sleep.

If this is the reason for poor sleep, anything that reduces stress may improve sleep. This can include relaxation, breathing and/or meditation techniques, certain yoga postures, healthy diet and lifestyle changes. We will look at some of these in a moment.

Melatonin is a natural hormone produced at night that helps regulate sleep/wake cycles. The right level of melatonin can help you sleep more deeply and lengthen your sleep cycle. If you get sleepy during the day even though you had plenty of rest, it's a sign that you have too much melatonin production. When the sun goes down and darkness occurs, the pineal gland, located just above the middle of the brain, is 'turned on' and begins to actively produce melatonin, which is released into the blood. Usually, this occurs around 9 pm. As a result, melatonin levels in the blood rise sharply and you begin to feel less alert as your body starts to prepare to sleep. Melatonin levels in the blood stay elevated for about 12 hours – all through the night – before the light of a new day when they fall back to low, barely detectable, daytime levels by about 9 am.

The natural production of melatonin to aid sleep patterns needs a person to be in a dimly lit setting. In addition to sunlight, artificial indoor lighting can be bright enough to prevent the release of melatonin. Several studies have showed that melatonin levels are diminished in people with Alzheimer's disease when compared with age-matched control subjects. Whether low melatonin is related to the cause or to the effect of Alzheimer's disease is still being researched but the severity of the symptoms of dementia has been proven to directly link to the decrease in nighttime melatonin levels.

So, in order to sleep well, we need to lower our stress level and to also achieve the right level of melatonin.

Bredesen (2014) recommends optimum sleep of eight hours per night and Perlmutter (2014) goes further, recommending that sleep patterns should be combined with eating patterns too. The last meal of the day should be eaten at least three hours before sleep, with eight hours of sleep and the next meal not to be eaten until 12 hours after the last meal. So, for example, if an evening meal is eaten at seven o'clock and sleep starts at ten thirty, you would wake up no earlier than six thirty in the morning and eat breakfast at seven o'clock.

The Sleep Foundation suggests a sleep hygiene programme that will help us to achieve this. Sleep hygiene is a range of practices that are necessary to quality nighttime sleep and daytime alertness.

A study in 2015 by P. Strøm-Tejsen and colleagues objectively measured the effects of bedroom air quality on sleep and next-day performance. The study highlights how it is often possible to select bedroom air temperature at will, but in bedrooms with the window closed for energy conservation and the internal door closed for privacy, the effective ventilation rate is often so poor that CO_2 levels routinely exceed 2500 ppm. This occurs in cold or temperate regions and certainly also in air-conditioned bedrooms in hot-humid regions. The study found that sleep quality improved significantly when the CO_2 level was lower, as did next-day reported sleepiness and ability to concentrate and the subjects' performance of a test of logical thinking. The simple and effective solution was to increase the clean outdoor air supply into the bedroom by opening the window.

Good practice for a good night's sleep

- **Avoid napping during the day** because it disturbs the normal pattern of sleep and wakefulness.

- **Exercise regularly** to build muscle mass and increase brain output of serotonin and dopamine, brain chemicals that reduce anxiety and depression.

- **Ensure adequate exposure to natural light.** This is particularly important for older people who may not venture outside often. Light exposure helps maintain a healthy sleep–wake cycle.

- **Keep your blood sugar stable.** Avoid sugar in the diet and refined carbohydrates to keep from spiking your insulin production. Keep well hydrated – dehydration puts the body in stress and raises cortisol levels. Keep pure water by your bed and drink it when you first wake up and before you go to sleep.

- **Establish a regular relaxing bedtime routine.** For example, set a habit of a warm bath, a warm drink, listening to relaxing music. Try to avoid emotionally upsetting conversations and activities before trying to go to sleep. Don't dwell on or bring your problems to bed.

- **Make sure the bedroom air quality is high and that the bedroom is pleasant and relaxing.** Open the window a small way, if the outside air is of high quality. Check the comfort of the bed and the pillow. Check that the room temperature is comfortable and that the light level is relaxing.

- **Consider anti-stress supplements** like B vitamins, minerals like calcium, magnesium, chromium and zinc, and antioxidants like vitamin C, alpha lipoic acid, grapeseed extract and CoQ10. Adaptogen herbs like ginseng, astragalus, eleuthero, schisandra, tulsi (holy basil), rhodiola and ashwagandha help the body cope with the side effects of stress and rebalance the metabolism. These supplement and herbs will not only lower cortisol levels but they will also help you decrease the effects of stress on the body by boosting the immune system.

Always check with your GP before you start any supplements.

Meditate and relax!

Most people now know and accept that meditation provides us with many benefits, including reduced tension and stress and improved focus and concentration. Studies are revealing that meditation could also lead to improvement in the brain's grey matter. Grey matter is another word for the cerebral cortex and, as a major component of the central nervous system, is found in areas of the brain involved in muscle control, seeing and hearing, memory, emotions, speech, decision-making and self-control.

A study at Massachusetts General Hospital, Harvard Medical School, USA, discovered that meditation increased the density of the grey matter within the hippocampus, a region of the brain important for learning and memory, and in structures associated with self-awareness, compassion and introspection.

Scans were taken at the beginning and end of the eight-week study. From the results, researchers determined that meditation literally rebuilds the brain's grey matter in just eight weeks, making this the very first study to document that meditation produces this kind of change over time. The changes observed in the meditators were not seen in the control group, signifying that they had not come about naturally over time, but rather that the daily act of meditating had produced them.

Participants also reported reductions in stress after the eight weeks, which makes sense, as over the course of the study, the grey-matter density in the amygdala – which is known to play an important role in stress and anxiety – decreased.

This study is groundbreaking, and empowering in that it shows that we have the power to change the structure of our own brains: to improve our memory and learning capacities and to become more compassionate and self-aware.

Britta Holzel, first author of the study, summarised its incredible findings: 'It is fascinating to see the brain's plasticity and that, by practicing meditation, we can play an active role in changing the brain and can increase our well-being and quality of life' (Holzel *et al.* 2011). You can also visit the TedTalk by Sara Lazar (2011), a neuroscientist also involved in this study, where she presents amazing brain scans showing that meditation changes the size of key regions of our brain. We will be exploring more about plasticity in the next chapter.

Another similar study by Eileen Luders and colleagues (2015) also found that there are potential age-defying effects of long-term meditation on grey matter.

Participants in the Holzel and colleagues (2011) study practised forms of mindfulness meditation every day for approximately 30 minutes. Mindfulness is a meditation style that emphasises maintaining an objective awareness of sensations, feelings and states of mind. Essentially, it is all about combining breathing techniques with paying attention to the present and not allowing the mind to wander to the past or the future.

Mindfulness meditation is usually practised sitting or lying with eyes closed and with the back straight. Attention is focused on one object or action. Initially, attention may be put on the movement of the abdomen when breathing in and out, or on the awareness of the breath as it goes in and out the nostrils. As thoughts come up, you should return to focusing on the object of meditation, such as the breathing. If you notice that your mind has wandered, you simply bring it back to the object of meditation. Meditators often start with short periods of 10 minutes or so a day. As you practise regularly, it becomes easier to keep the attention focused on breathing.

With practice, awareness of the breath can be extended into mindful awareness of thoughts, feelings and actions.

There are many published guides to mindfulness meditation in book or electronic format. YouTube is a good source of guided mindfulness exercises, including an excellent 20 minute one by Jeremy Woodall (2013) that will get you started.

Exercise to your heart's and brain's content

You will have noticed that exercise has been mentioned more than once so far in this chapter. Leading a physically active lifestyle can have a significant impact on well-being and it is well documented that exercise is beneficial for physical and mental health, with recent studies showing that exercise may improve memory and slow down mental decline. In fact, the Alzheimer's Society (2015) suggests that taking regular physical exercise appears to be one of the best things that you can do to reduce your risk of getting a condition that causes dementia.

They combined the results of 11 studies to show that regular exercise can significantly reduce the risk of developing symptoms of dementia by about 30 per cent. For Alzheimer's disease specifically, the risk was reduced by 45 per cent.

One particular study, known as the Caerphilly Cohort Study and funded by the Medical Research Council, Alzheimer's Society and the British Heart Foundation, looked at health behaviours of over 2000 men in Wales, and followed them for 35 years (Elwood *et al.* 2013). Of the five behaviours that were assessed (regular exercise, not smoking, moderate alcohol intake, healthy body weight and healthy diet), exercise had the greatest effect in terms of reducing dementia risk. Overall, people who followed four or five of the above behaviours were up to 60 per cent less likely to develop symptoms of dementia. This is compelling information for following the lifestyle recommendations I have described in this book.

Exercise affects the brain on multiple fronts. It increases heart rate, which pumps more oxygen to the brain. It also aids the bodily release of several hormones, all of which participate in aiding and providing a nourishing environment for brain cells.

Exercise stimulates the brain plasticity by stimulating growth of new connections between cells in a wide range of important cortical areas of the brain. Research by Molteni and colleagues (2004) from UCLA demonstrated that exercise increased growth factors in the brain, making it easier for the brain to grow new neuronal connections.

From a behavioural perspective, the same antidepressant-like effects associated with 'runner's high' found in humans are associated with a drop in stress hormones. A study (Bjornebekk, Mathe and Brene 2005) from Stockholm showed that the antidepressant effect of running was also associated with more cell growth in the hippocampus, an area of the brain responsible for learning and memory.

What does 'exercise' mean?

The research studies in this area do not all use the same definition of 'physical activity' or exercise. In general, they are referring to aerobic exercise performed for a sustained period. The Department of Exercise Science at the University of Georgia suggests that as little as 20 minutes of exercise will improve information processing and memory functions.

Physical exercise does not just mean playing a sport or running. It can also mean a daily activity such as brisk walking, cleaning or gardening. And of course, it can include leisure activities such as dancing and even shopping. Even if you, your family member or friend is frail, it is possible to take part in seated physical activity that will boost heart and brain health.

Consider, too, where the physical activity takes place. Researchers from the University of Essex (Barton and Pretty 2010) found that as little as five minutes of a 'green activity' such as walking, gardening, cycling or farming can boost mood and self-esteem. 'We believe that there would be a large potential benefit to individuals, society and to the costs of the health service if all groups of people were to self-medicate more with green exercise', Barton said in a statement about the study, which was published in the journal *Environmental Science and Technology*.

Many studies have shown that outdoor exercise can reduce the risk of mental illness and improve a sense of well-being, but Jules Pretty and Jo Barton, who led this study, said that until now no one knew how much time needed to be spent on green exercise for the benefits to show. Barton and Pretty looked at data from 1252 people of different ages, genders and mental health status, taken from 10 existing studies in Britain. They found that the largest positive effect on self-esteem came from a five-minute dose of 'green exercise'.

All natural environments were beneficial, including parks in towns or cities, they said, but green areas with water appeared to have a more positive effect.

In summary, this chapter has set out the current thinking about emotion and how what you feel affects your brain.

What you feel is impacted on by relationships and interactions with others. What you feel is also a result and a cause of how tense or relaxed you are. Again, this is likely to be a result of those connections with others but also is a result of your own ability to control the emotions that give rise to those feelings.

For an individual who is experiencing cognitive difficulties, these abilities to connect with others, control behaviour in response to emotions and even to get a good night's sleep can be impaired. The downward spiral into worsening symptoms of dementia then begins as distressed feelings lead to distressed behaviour, which is misunderstood and negatively responded to by others. This undermining interaction leads to yet more distress, distressed behaviour and further symptoms of dementia. That spiral can only end up as a devastating self-fulfilling negative experience for all.

But the good news is that, as you have seen, all of these factors are within our own control. As with nutrition, the important and exciting message is that we can do something to improve our brain function by addressing those emotional states and use a framework to help the person exercise and to get a good night's sleep. So, it is possible to reduce the symptoms of dementia in those who are living with the disability.

I hope that this chapter has highlighted for you how you can support the person you know to sleep, relax and to connect with you and others as further approaches to cognitive rehabilitation and rementia.

Chapter 6

Cognitive Rehabilitation

*Cognition, or How What You
Do Affects Your Brain*

When a clinician refers to cognition or cognitive processes they are referring to how individuals think, perceive, remember, judge and learn. These processes involve higher-level functions of the brain that control language, imagination, perception and planning.

Immediately you can see that therefore the broad term of 'memory problems' is in fact not helpful in understanding the symptoms of dementia and the cognitive impairments a person is experiencing and how to overcome these.

Memory is just one cognitive function and even that is more complex than the simple taking in, storing and recalling of pieces of information. I'm going to show you some of the most common types of memory function and how knowledge of these can help with a rehabilitation approach to improving each of them.

Short-term memory

Initially, new information is held in short-term memory, which is not really 'memory' at all but actually the temporary ability to hold a few pieces of information just long enough to use them. The duration of short-term memory is believed to be between 15 and 30 seconds and the number of elements that can be held thought to be between five and nine.

Some evidence supports the concept that short-term memory depends upon electrical and chemical events in the brain as opposed to structural changes, such as the formation of new synapses. After a period of time, information may be moved into a more permanent type of memory, long-term memory, which is the result of anatomical or biochemical changes that occur in the brain.

So when many people describe someone with dementia as having 'short-term memory problems' and then go on to define this as the person being unable to remember what they had for dinner the previous evening, what they really mean is that the person has difficulty in moving that information into a more permanent, long-term memory (in other words a difficulty with new learning).

A true representation of the sort of difficulty that someone with short-term memory may have is, for example, when they cannot hold the topic of a conversation in their head while they are engaging in it. Or they cannot hold a fact, such as a telephone number, while they operate the phone to make a call.

It is important to distinguish the type of memory difficulty that a person has so that you can then try to overcome that particular problem.

Working memory

Psychologists use the term 'working memory' to describe the ability we have to hold in mind and mentally manipulate information; this includes drawing on previous memories too in order to problem solve. Working memory is often thought of as a mental workspace that we can use to store important information in the course of our mental activities. The main difference between short-term and working memory is therefore the ability to manipulate information.

Long-term memory

Permanent long-term memories can also be sub-divided into different types and it is helpful to understand these so that if you or a person you are supporting has a difficulty with one type you can work on compensating for or restoring that function.

Episodic memory

This is the memory for important or significant episodes in the person's life. They often have a strong sensation or a strong emotion attached to them that serve to keep the memory vivid and accessible to the person. Positive episodic memories can be used to reminisce with the person and will support brain stimulation, communication and stress reduction. Individuals who support and care for a person who is living with dementia must also be aware of episodic memories that relate to negative feelings so that they can support the person through these feelings, using their emotional intelligence and the person-centred approaches described in Chapter 5.

Semantic memory

This refers to general world knowledge (facts, ideas, meaning and concepts) that we have accumulated throughout our lives. It refers to general facts and meanings that can be shared with others, whereas episodic memory refers to unique personal experiences. Semantic memory, particularly more recent memory that has been accumulated, may be lost, whilst the individual might still able to hold onto more remote, well-rehearsed semantic memories. So names of grandchildren and extended family members may be more difficult to remember than the name of a well-loved family pet who has long since died.

Recent research has focused on the idea that when people access a word's meaning, sensorimotor information that is used to perceive and act on the object that the word suggests is automatically activated. This supports the idea that the meaning of a particular word is grounded in the sensorimotor systems. For example, when you think of an orange, your knowledge of it is in multiple sensory images of smell, texture, colour and taste. As you have seen, each of these sensory functions is within a different area of the brain's cortex. So, an individual can 'know' an orange through a single or multiple sensory image recognition. In other words, you can know an orange with your eyes closed just from its taste, smell or feel.

This is important information when you are supporting a person who is living with dementia because, if they have lost their ability to recognise an object through one sense, you can present it to them through one or more of the other four senses and, if those cognitive areas are still intact, the person will still be able to recognise and engage with that object.

Procedural memory

This is the memory for the ways of doing an activity (the process). Rather than being stored in brain cell connections, procedural memories are actually stored in the familiar pattern of movements that have become a well-rehearsed skill.

Many everyday activities use procedural memory: driving, running upstairs, making a cup of tea in a familiar kitchen, getting dressed.

A good example of an activity that uses procedural memory is learning to drive. To begin with, we use our working memory to hold the driving instructions (mirror, signal, manoeuvre; declutch to change gear; declutch and brake at the same time). This kind of complex mental activity in which we have to both keep in mind some information while processing other material requires working memory ability.

As we rehearse the same activity over time, we no longer need to hold the information in mind unless a new decision connected to the activity needs to be made or a problem needs to be solved. Otherwise, we are able to act on the 'muscle memory' of procedural memory. Procedural memory allows us to carry out actions that are retained in the process of doing something (motor actions) without needing to consciously think about them. Clearly, this form of memory performance might still be accessible by people with dementia who have lost their explicit skills of working memory or semantic memory.

Supporting individuals to be more able by accessing their procedural memories relies on others to create the environment for this. So, for example, a person might not be able to learn a new route to the bathroom from the bed but they might be able to use their well-established procedural memory to take a familiar route if the bed is placed in the same position in relationship to the bathroom door as it was in their previous or a well-remembered place of residence.

Prospective memory

This is the memory for what needs to be done in the future and can range from appointments to remembering to turn off the gas hob. Most of us use a range of trusted methods to hold onto prospective memories, often with the use of simple technology such as an oven timer, a calendar, post-it notes and apps. These same methods can be useful to an individual with dementia, although the use of some of these may rely initially on a new learning pattern in order to use them effectively.

Stages of dementia and levels of ability

All conditions that cause dementia are progressive and will increasingly damage the structure and chemistry of the brain over time. How quickly the symptoms of dementia progress depends on many inter-related factors including physical make-up, emotional resilience and the support available to the person. Viewing dementia as a series of stages can be a useful way to understand the illness, but it is important to realise that this only provides a rough guide to the progress of the condition. The Alzheimer's Society in the UK describes the progression in three stages: early, middle and later.

They describe the early stages of dementia as being when a person's symptoms will be noticeable and will affect their day-to-day life. However, someone in the early stages of dementia will be fairly independent and should be able to do most things with a little help, or perhaps a little differently. In the middle stage the person will need more support to help them to manage their day-to-day life. They are likely to become increasingly forgetful, particularly of names, and may sometimes repeat the same question or sentence over and over. They may also fail to recognise people or confuse them with others. At this stage, the person might put themselves or others at risk through their forgetfulness, for example by not lighting the gas on the cooker or forgetting to take medication.

The later stage usually describes someone who is likely to be much frailer and be reliant on others for much of their care.

A person in the later stages is likely to experience severe memory loss, problems with communication and daily activities, and greater changes in behaviour and physical problems than in the earlier stages.

Whilst this delineation of dementia can be helpful for determining, for example, the level of care that a person needs, it can also be misleading as individuals can fluctuate in their abilities depending on their physical and emotional health and the physical and emotional environment that they find themselves in. The risk of viewing dementia as a progression of stages is that it creates an expectation of a downward spiral with no opportunity for maintaining abilities for longer.

I developed my PAL Instrument in 1999 with the encouragement and mentorship of Professor Tom Kitwood because I was convinced that a more helpful view of dementia is to identify the ability level of each individual. With that viewpoint, we are likely to enable rather than disable the person as we understand the physical and social environment required to sustain those abilities. If we only recognise the difficulties an individual is having, we will always disable them as we will only provide care and support to address their difficulties. So, the PAL Instrument uses a strengths-based approach, underpinned by cognitive developmental theory.

The PAL (short for Pool Activity Level) has a Checklist of statements that identifies how the person can perform in nine everyday activities. There are four statements for each of the activities and each statement describes a slightly different level of ability. By completing the PAL Checklist, it is possible to identify the overall level of cognitive and functional ability and, using that knowledge, to select the appropriate PAL Profile which describes how to support the person at that level of ability.

The four levels of ability are:

Planned activity level

At a planned activity level the person can work towards completing an activity, but may not be able to solve any problems that arise while in the process. He or she will be able to look in obvious places for equipment needed but may not be able to search beyond the usual places. A caregiver assisting someone at this level will need to keep their sentences short, and to avoid using words like 'and' or 'but' which tend to be used to link two sentences together into a more complex one. Caregivers will also need to stand by to help solve any problems should they arise. People functioning at a planned activity level are able to carry out activities that achieve a tangible result.

Exploratory activity level

At an exploratory activity level, the person can carry out very familiar activities in familiar surroundings. He or she will find objects that are needed to carry out the activity only if these are in their line of vision. So, objects need to be out of cupboards and in view. At this level people are more concerned with the effect of doing the activity than with the consequence and may not have an end result in mind. Therefore, a creative and spontaneous approach to activities from caregivers is helpful. If an activity involves more than two or three steps, a person at this level will need help in breaking the activity into manageable chunks. Directions need to be made very simple and the use of memory aids such as task lists, calendars and labelling of frequently used items can be very helpful.

Sensory activity level

At a sensory activity level, the person may not have many thoughts or ideas about carrying out an activity; he or she is mainly concerned with sensation and with moving his or her body in response to those sensations. He or she will only find objects that are within arm's reach, so things need to be placed where they can be easily accessed. People at this level can be guided to carry out single step activities such as sweeping or winding wool. More complex activities can only be carried out when directed one step at a time. Therefore, caregivers need to ensure that the person at this activity level has the opportunity to experience a wide variety of sensations, and to carry out one step activities. Directions to maximise this opportunity need to be kept very simple and to be reinforced by demonstrating the action required.

Reflex activity level

A person at a reflex activity level may not be aware of the surrounding environment or even of his or her own body. He or she is living in a subliminal or sub-conscious state, where movement is a reflex response to a stimulus. Therefore, people wishing to enter into this person's consciousness need to use direct sensory stimulation and place objects so that they touch the reflex 'zones' of the palm of the hand, the foot or the face. By using direct stimulation to these areas, reflex responses of grasping, toe spreading or curling and mouth opening will take place. Doing so is a way of recognising and nurturing the ability of the person and can potentially raise their level of self-awareness. A person at this level may have difficulty in organising more than one sensation which is being experienced at the same time. Excessive or multiple stimuli can cause distress, therefore crowds, loud noises and background clamour should be avoided. Activities at this level should focus on introducing a single sensation to the person. A caregiver interacting with a person at a reflex level needs to use all their communication skills to enter into the world of the person. Language skills tend to play only a minor role and should be kept to single word directions, although the use of facial expression and of a warm and reassuring tone and volume can be vital in establishing a communication channel.

In 2008, the PAL Instrument Checklist was validated by Jennifer Wenborn and team at the Department of Mental Health Sciences, University College London. It is translated into several languages and is now used within research programmes and also in health and social care settings to support care and activity planning. The PAL Checklist and four PAL Profiles are found in the Appendix and you are free to use them to inform your Rementia Plan for yourself or the person whom you are supporting.

Using the PAL Instrument and understanding your own specific memory difficulties and symptoms of dementia or those of the person you care for will enable you to plan how to improve brain function and to reduce the symptoms of dementia through cognitive rehabilitation therapy (CRT) and cognitive stimulation therapy (CST).

Cognitive stimulation therapy

Cognitive stimulation works on the 'use it or lose it' principle and is achieved by supporting the person to engage through all of their senses in a range of preferred activities that will systematically target the main cognitive functions including thinking, reasoning, perception and judgement.

Examples of cognitive stimulation activities include:

- movement to music

- current affairs discussion

- newspaper photo discussion

- number games

- throw and catch

- word games

- creative activity

- sensory activities – touch, smell, taste, hearing, sight.

So, CST is a well-established group psychosocial intervention for people with dementia. It offers a range of enjoyable activities providing general stimulation for thinking, concentration and memory in a social small group setting. Its roots can be traced back to reality orientation (RO), which was developed in the late 1950s as a response to confusion and disorientation in older patients in hospital units in the USA. Cognitive stimulation is often discussed in normal ageing as well as in dementia. This reflects a general view that lack of cognitive activity hastens cognitive decline. With people with dementia, cognitive stimulation attempts to make use of the positive aspects of RO whilst ensuring that the stimulation is implemented in a sensitive, respectful and person-centred manner.

In 2017, Professor Martin Orrell and his colleagues published the results of their research study into the effectiveness of CST as a home-based programme of cognitive stimulation delivered by family caregivers. This study aimed to evaluate the effectiveness of a home-based, caregiver-led individual cognitive stimulation therapy (iCST) programme in improving cognition and quality of life (QoL) for the person with dementia and mental and physical health (well-being) for the caregiver.

The results were that there was no evidence that iCST has an effect on cognition or quality of life for people with dementia. However, participating in iCST appeared to enhance the quality of the caregiving relationship and caregivers' quality of life.

It was suggested that more tailored approaches might have greater effects and cognitive rehabilitation therapy is one of the approaches that was being researched at the same time.

Cognitive rehabilitation therapy

Cognitive rehabilitation therapy is the process of improving functional ability that has been lost or altered as a result of damage to brain cells/chemistry. If skills cannot be relearned, then new ones are taught to enable the person to compensate for their lost cognitive functions. Whilst in this book I have been describing all approaches to nutrition, emotional health and brain function as forms of cognitive rehabilitation, CRT is usually taken to mean the individualised programme of specific skills training and practice.

The research work, led by Professor Linda Clare at the University of Exeter (2008, p.93), has identified that there are some basic principles for cognitive rehabilitation therapy:

- It needs to include a focus on emotional responses (loss, anger, fear, frustration, anxiety) and take into account the impact on the person and their family.

- It needs to be goal driven – focus on the aspects of daily life which are of concern to the person and their family.

- Interventions need to be based on the cognitive functioning profile of the individual – recognising their strengths and limitations.

- It is essential to understand the coping strategies of the individual – what works for them? Are they acknowledging the difficulties they have?

- It needs a collaborative approach with the person with dementia, their family carers and professionals.

- The outcomes must be monitored, evaluated and revised if needed.

For CRT to be effective, meaningful personal goals need to be selected by the individual and then the evidence-based rehabilitation strategies can be used to bring about improved functioning

Setting meaningful personal goals

There are many research papers that identify the importance of setting personally meaningful goals as central to the success of rehabilitation therapy. Wade (2009) reviewed several articles on this topic and concluded that working towards some elements of SMART (specific, measurable, achievable, realistic and time specific) goals will enhance performance. Not only does having a goal motivate the recipient of the therapy, it also clarifies for those providing the support what is being aimed for and helps to identify when it has been achieved.

Some examples of therapy goals that were formulated in the GREAT trial (Clare *et al.* 2013) led by Professor Linda Clare were:

- I will find my spectacles every time without asking my wife.

- I will learn to Skype with my grandson once a week.

- I will take my keys with me whenever I go out.

- I will be able to say the names of my grandchildren.

- I will be able to call my husband from my mobile phone.

As I have already discussed, a person might be having difficulty in achieving the stated goal for a number of reasons which could relate to their cognitive and physical ability, to the support of others and to the complexity of the activity itself.

So, for example, the finding of spectacles can be an issue of:

- attention difficulty – not noticing where you have put them

- memory storage – not storing the information about where you have put them

- recall – not remembering where you have put them

- perception – not recognising them

- visual impairment – not being able to see them

- reliance on others (learned helplessness).

Understanding the reasons for the difficulty is the first step to coming up with appropriate strategies and to devising an effective CRT plan. There is a range of approaches to support new learning and relearning lost skills and I will describe these strategies in two broad groups: Compensatory and Restorative.

Cognitive rehabilitation therapy: Compensatory strategies

The compensatory approach aim is to modify the demand an activity places on the person. This can be achieved in a number of ways:

- Simplifying the activity to remove or decrease the demand on the impaired ability, for example using ready-meals instead of cooking from scratch or setting up direct debits rather than having to remember to pay bills.

- Using memory aids and assistive technology, such as lists, calendars, white board notes, kitchen timers, electronic reminders.

- Creating helpful environments, such as keeping morning medication next to the toothbrush or placing a key hook next to the door so that the key isn't left in the lock but can easily be found.

Simplifying the activity

Coming up with alternatives to an activity that is becoming difficult to complete is an attractive option that will reduce frustration, reliance on others and possibly embarrassment. If you or the person you care for is not too worried about being able to continue to carry out an activity, this approach is a good idea and many people come up with ingenious solutions that work for them. However, if it is important to the person to be able to continue with the activity as it has always been done, then it may be better to try a restorative cognitive rehabilitation therapy approach that aims to relearn the lost skill. For example, if the person's sense of identity is strongly connected to being a home-maker and cook, it might undermine him or her even further if the role is reduced by relying on ready-meals and the better solution might be to relearn to make some favourite dishes.

Using memory aids and assistive technology

There are many memory aids that we all rely on to support our busy lives and these may support a person in the early stage of living with dementia.

Technology offers huge potential benefits for people with dementia, whether it's a familiar gadget such as a mobile phone and TV or a specific telecare device to remind someone to take medication. The UK Alzheimer's Society (2014) has developed a Dementia-friendly Technology Charter that gives people with dementia and their carers information on how to access this technology. The Charter also provides guidance to health, housing and social care professionals on how to make technology work for people based on their individual needs.

The overall aims of the Charter are:

- to help every person with dementia have the opportunity to benefit from technology appropriate to their needs

- to outline and encourage the implementation of high level principles and best practice for organisations that provide services to people with dementia.

Creating helpful environments

Combining already well-established routines with a new activity can be a very successful way of supporting new learning. This method is relying on your current procedural memory for a habitual activity that has been rehearsed so often that it has become part of your routine or pattern of doing something. By placing the new element of learning into the current routine, you are more likely first to notice it and second to add it into your habit through repetition, without having to cognitively learn and remember it. In other words, you are effectively bypassing the cognitive learning process and supporting the gaining of the skill through movement.

Equally, if you or the person you care for needs to break a habit and 'unlearn' something that is no longer helpful, you can apply the same principle and add a new sensory experience that interrupts the familiar routine and causes the person to notice what they are doing. For example, in the University of Exeter GREAT study, we had a participant who locked his door and left the key in the lock (as he had always done) and this meant that his carer could not get into the house in the morning. The solution that we introduced successfully was to add a small fluffy ball to the key ring and this worked by making him become aware of the key rather than acting automatically.

So you can see that environments can be helpful or bewildering because of the way that they are recognised. If you or the person you care for has perception difficulties, particularly making sense of what is seen or heard, you can adapt the environment both by controlling what is experienced, for example, background noise, and with the use of colour and helpful signage.

Auditory figure–ground discrimination problems arise when the person cannot pick out single sounds from background noise. For the individual, it must seem as though they are being bombarded with noise – no wonder they might be distressed or cannot concentrate on a conversation or an activity. The simple solution is to reduce as much background noise as possible, turning off the TV or radio but also allowing yourself to listen for other noises that you might have been filtering out without even realising it.

Visual perception refers to the brain's ability to make sense of what the eyes see. Visual figure–ground discrimination is one of the building blocks of visual perception and enables us to locate something in a busy or a same colour/pattern background. Good visual figure–ground discrimination skills are important for many everyday skills such as dining, dressing, using a TV remote or a telephone keypad.

Compensatory approaches to support this skill include simplifying the background so that objects become more visible. This can be done by reducing excessive patterns in backgrounds (such as carpets, seating and bed covers) and by having strong colour contrasts that help objects to clearly stand out.

The same principle can be applied to supporting the person to be able to use a TV remote or a keypad by placing a colourful raised dot on the most useful button and setting up the system so that minimal buttons need to be pressed. The Royal National Institute for the Blind (RNIB), for example, produces small tactile bright orange dots to mark the keys on a computer or typewriter keyboard, central heating or hi-fi controls.[1]

Notices, signage and 'land mark' objects that support you or the person to make sense of their environment can be very helpful if orientation, or way-finding, skills are being lost. Landmark objects can include coloured doors, pictures, furniture or ornaments indoors or buildings, pubs, shops, churches and post boxes outdoors. Highly visible indoor objects can be used to link to finding a smaller one, for example, learning to always put the house key next to an ornament on a shelf. Outdoor objects will need to be learned as part of a route and so also require some element of restorative approach to draw attention to them and embed the new learning.

Labels, notices and signs are most helpful if the font is strongly contrasting with the background and if the font is clear and easy to read. Lower case writing is easier to read than all upper case 'block' letters. This is because, once we have learned how to read and have become good at it, we tend to read by recognising the pattern of the word rather than by working out the combination of letters. A word that is written in lower case (e.g. Toilet) will have a more distinctive pattern than one that is written in capitals (e.g. TOILET). Written signs that include a picture of the object help to illustrate and add more visual meaning. So, in the example of the Toilet sign, it would be most helpful to have a picture of a toilet rather than the more traditional picture of a stick person.

---

1   http://shop.rnib.org.uk/loc-dots-orange.html

You can find more information about creating helpful environments through colour and design in my book, published by the Alzheimer's Society in 2015, *Alzheimer's Society Guide to the Dementia Care Environment*. The reference and link to the ebook is in the reading list at the end of this book.

Whilst all three of the compensatory approaches described here are focusing not on restoring lost function but rather on modifying the activity, it is likely that there will be an element of still needing to acquire some new learning and both compensatory and restorative approaches may be used together. For example, the person may use a coloured bump on the TV remote but they still need to learn what the button is for and possibly the sequence that needs to be followed.

Cognitive rehabilitation therapy: Restorative strategies

Restorative strategies are designed to restore lost function through regular practice of the activity using techniques that address the cognitive impairment that is causing the functional difficulty. So, the first question when designing a cognitive rehabilitation plan is: 'What is the cognitive impairment that is getting in the way of carrying out the activity?' You have already seen examples of this in the previous chapters where I have shown you how different cognitive impairments can each be causing a difficulty in carrying out an activity such as dining or communication and how different compensatory solutions might help.

It is important to understand that the restorative programme is not aiming to cure the cause of the dementia symptom or to improve the cognitive impairment, and so success is not measured by the scores on a cognitive test. The aim is to make use of the brain's ability for reorganisation (termed plasticity) and support a new network of brain cell connections to be made in place of the damaged ones. Therefore, success is measured by an improvement in the ability to carry out an action, although the method of doing so may be different from the previous way you or the person did this

The three guiding principles to successful cognitive rehabilitation therapy restorative strategies are:

- learn from success and not from mistakes (errorless learning)

- making the brain work hard will make the brain work (effortful processing)

- presenting information through all of the senses will help in learning and recall (multi-modal support).

Errorless learning

Errorless learning is a technique that reduces or eliminates errors during learning. It is the opposite of 'trial and error learning'. If you or the person is exposed to making a mistake this might be what is remembered rather than the correct way of carrying out the activity. So, the therapeutic technique is to break down the activity into smaller, achievable steps and then to gradually put these together as success at each step is achieved.

In 2013, Maartje Me de Werd and colleagues published a research paper about the effectiveness of errorless learning of everyday tasks in people with dementia. She and her colleagues found that this approach is effective in teaching adults with dementia a variety of meaningful daily tasks or skills, with gains being generally maintained at follow-up. They showed that individuals with dementia are still able to acquire meaningful skills and engage in worthwhile activities, which may potentially increase their autonomy and independence, and ultimately their quality of life, as well as reduce caregiver burden and professional dependency.

The errorless learning approach uses these principles:

- **No guessing**: The person is encouraged not to guess to prevent errors. Either the correct response is immediately offered, after which the participant is asked to repeat it, or the correct response is provided in case of hesitation or uncertainty.

- **Stepwise approach**: The activity is broken down into steps and is mastered one step at a time. If the person cannot manage a step they are immediately shown the correct way and they are encouraged to begin again at a step they can manage.

- **Modelling**: The helper demonstrates to the person how each step is to be performed. The person is first invited to repeat and master each step, before he/she is asked to execute the whole activity unprompted, independently and without errors.

- **Verbal instruction**: It is explicitly explained to the person what to do in each of the activity steps or what is to be repeated. The person is regularly reminded that, if they are not sure of an answer, either to say 'I'm not sure' or just not to respond. When this occurs, the person is immediately provided with a cue or prompt to assist them in recalling the correct answer.

- **Visual instruction**: The helper gives the person a visual cue or prompt to help guide them through the activity, such as a checklist with pictograms, a written action plan, or coloured stickers to indicate a specific object or place.

- **Vanishing cues**: Targets are presented and cues gradually withheld after successful recall trials until the person is able to give the correct response in the absence of cues.

Effortful processing

Memory is an information processing system in three stages: encoding, storage and retrieval of information. We get information into our brains through a process called encoding, which is the input of information into the memory system. Once we receive sensory information from the environment, our brains label or code it. We organise the information with other similar information and connect new concepts to existing concepts. Encoding information occurs through automatic processing and effortful processing.

Different levels of information require either automatic or effortful processing, depending on the complexity of the information, the ability of the individual and the meaningfulness of the information to the person. For someone who is living with the symptoms of dementia, automatic processing becomes less possible and, in order to learn and recall information, effortful processing with a focus of attention and conscious effort is needed.

Effortful processing is supported by giving fewer prompts so that the person makes the highest effort to learn and retrieve information. Research by Professor Linda Clare (2008, p.97) at the University of Exeter shows that low-effort conditions where the person is given the answer immediately or given a lot of prompting is not supportive of new learning and cognitive rehabilitation. To assist in encoding information through effortful processing, it is helpful to elaborate on the item by associating it with images or related meanings. Cues are more effective when they have meaning.

Even a simple sentence is easier to recall when it is meaningful. Read the following sentences (Bransford and McCarrell 1974), then look away and count backwards in threes from 30 to zero, and then try to write down the sentences (no peeking back at this page!):

- The notes were sour because the seams split.

- The voyage wasn't delayed because the bottle shattered.

- The haystack was important because the cloth ripped.

How well did you do? By themselves, the statements that you wrote down were most likely confusing and difficult for you to recall. Now, try writing them again, using the following prompts: bagpipe, ship christening and parachutist. Next count backwards from 40 by fours, then check yourself to see how well you recalled the sentences this time. You can see that the sentences are now much more memorable because each of the sentences was placed in context. Material is far better encoded when you make it meaningful.

Multi-modal support

Multi-sensory experiences during the cognitive rehabilitation therapy restorative activity can be beneficial in encoding and later recalling what has been learned. Examples include the use of sounds, smells, colour or texture to add to the activity experience.

There are three main ways in which information can be encoded: visual (picture), acoustic (sound) and semantic (meaning). Information is detected by the sense organs and enters the sensory memory. If attended to, this information enters the short-term memory and then transfers to the long-term memory only if that information is rehearsed (i.e. repeated). So, providing the person with the opportunity to repeatedly experience the information in a consistent way, through the range of their senses, gives them more opportunity to hold onto that information.

If maintenance rehearsal (repetition) does not occur, then information is forgotten, and lost from short-term memory through the processes of displacement or decay. This brings us to the technique for rehearsing the information or action in order to transfer it into the long-term semantic, episodic, procedural or perspective types of memory. Please do take a look back at the start of this chapter to remind yourself of these different types of long-term memory (see pages 85–88)).

There are several tried and tested rehabilitation techniques that can be combined with the approaches of errorless learning, effortful processing and multi-modal support. It is difficult to guide you here to which technique you should select to support the person in their cognitive rehabilitation restorative therapy because individuals are very different and it will depend on a range of factors, including their impairment, ability, preferences and motivation. People are not like cars and do not come with a manual that guides us how to 'fix' them. However, Table 6.1 below will give you some helpful starting points.

Expanding rehearsal

Expanding rehearsal is a technique that helps to retain information. This strategy is beneficial for learning facts and for practising the process of doing an activity as it helps the person to gradually build up their knowledge or skill with spaced practice. The helper blends this technique with the errorless learning approach, providing the correct response when the person hesitates or indicates that they don't know the correct response. The recall interval is then reduced until the person is able to reproduce the desired response, after which the interval is increased again until the person is able to give the correct response after the longest interval.

Expanding rehearsal is useful for factual learning, such as face–name associations, object naming, memory for object location and prospective memory assignments. The person is supported to practise recalling facts at gradually expanding intervals.

The aim is to remember one thing and test your memory of this at small time intervals. So, for example, you read the name of your new granddaughter 'Grace' and then test whether you remember it 30 seconds later. You then double the time between saying the name and remembering it: one minute, two minutes, four minutes, eight minutes, 16 minutes and 32 minutes. You must get it right to move onto the next time period. If not, remind yourself by looking at the written name and start again.

The goal is mastered when the information is successfully recalled at the final time-point of 32 minutes which is when, typically, a goal can be mastered. You will see that this means that the goal will have been intensively practised seven times in just over one hour.

Practice sessions occur within the context of a situation that provides social interaction, such as a casual conversation.

Expanding rehearsal can also be used for carrying out the process of an activity by gradually expanding the time between practice sessions. This can be used for process learning, such as using a TV remote, accessing phone messages or making a hot drink. More complex activities will be broken into smaller manageable steps and then the person is supported to practise each step of the activity at gradually expanding intervals. This is called 'chunking'.

Chunking and cueing

Chunking facts or steps in the process of an activity by putting them into categories or small groups can be helpful. Organising information into small, relevant, simple chunks or categories means that there is less information to remember. This technique supports the way that our brains naturally encode and store information. Think of it as being a little like a filing cabinet or a book shelf with folders on it; or a computer system of files and sub-folders.

To carry out an activity, break it down into single steps and then chunk them gradually, adding each step until the whole activity is achieved. Each time another step is added, practise the combination of steps with the expanding rehearsal approach until those steps have been mastered before adding the next step.

An example of using this natural approach as a focused therapy technique is the practice of making a grocery list by chunking items based on their locations in the supermarket or in the kitchen at home: fruit and vegetables, dairy, meat, canned goods, cleaning products, etc. The items can then be rehearsed, using the expanding rehearsal technique, so that the list is not relied on.

To support the rehearsal method, the recall of the list items can be cued by adding number associations: five fruit and vegetables items, three dairy, two meat, etc., or by letters of the alphabet: three beginning with 'B' (bread, butter, bananas), two beginning with 'M' (mince and mushrooms), etc.

This is only an example and the techniques of chunking and cueing can be applied to many activities. However, the activity must be meaningful to the person. So, in the example above, they must want to be able to remember items at the shop. Otherwise it would be better for them to simply use the list.

Cueing can also be used as a conversational technique to support recall without giving the person the full information. So, a helper could give the person information to help them remember something in particular, for example, to help orientate them to which restaurant they are going to for dinner with cues such as 'It's the white building by the sea, we went there with Jack and Elizabeth last time'.

Mnemonics

Useful mnemonics strategies include linking visual imagery, stories, poems or acronyms to the information to be remembered. For example, when I was a child, I was taught the mnemonic: **R**ichard **O**f **Y**ork **G**ave **B**attle **I**n **V**ain as a method of learning and recalling the colours of the rainbow in order: **R**ed, **O**range, **Y**ellow, **G**reen, **B**lue, **I**ndigo, **V**iolet.

More recently, I was illustrating this strategy in a conference presentation and used the mnemonic: **M**y **V**ery **E**nergetic **M**onkey **J**umps over the **SUN** to illustrate the planets in our solar system: **M**ercury, **V**enus, **E**arth, **M**ars, **J**upiter, **S**aturn, **U**ranus, **N**eptune! And I added to my presentation slide a picture of the sun and an animation of a monkey jumping over it. This visual imagery added to the factual information helped to make it more memorable and when the group was given repeated opportunity during the presentation to recall the order of the planets in increasing time frames (expanding rehearsal), they were able to retain the information and recall it the following day.

Prompting (and fading out of prompts)

Providing reminders of an action at strategic points of an activity can help to ensure success. Helpers can provide the prompts initially and then aim to reduce how often they are required. For example, when learning to use the calendar to find out the date, the helper will prompt the person to look at the calendar rather than answer a question about the date or an appointment themselves. In time they will need to prompt the person less, as checking the calendar will become habit.

Prompting to alert the person to attend to a sensory cue is helpful for those with an impairment of their attention ability. Alerting language includes simple words spoken with increased tone and emotion according to the specific situation. For example: 'Oh, look!', 'My goodness, listen to this!', 'Wow! Smell this!', 'Watch this!'. When combined with some appropriate touch, such as a hand on the shoulder or forearm, the person is supported to pay attention to the cue and therefore is more able to encode the information – the first step to creating a new memory.

Reality orientation

Reality orientation is an approach that aims to improve cognitive functioning and communication in individuals with dementia by using repetition and a range of resources such as clocks and calendars to help the memory. It involves regularly reminding the person of such information as the time, date, where he/she is and planned events for that day, such as a visit to see a friend. It is based on the belief that continually and repeatedly telling or showing certain reminders to people with mild to moderate memory loss will result in an increase in interaction with others and improved orientation. This, in turn, can improve self-esteem.

Reality orientation can be used to assist an individual with dementia towards an awareness of the 'here and now', by offering reminders of the day, date, etc. regularly throughout the day. These reminders can be provided verbally or through activities and visual prompts, such as diaries and calendars. Some individuals with dementia may benefit from regular access to a board for them to refer to (such as a pin board or white board) which contains up-to-date information about their day.

A person-centred use of reality orientation aims to raise individuals' awareness of where they are in time and place, and of who they are. In conversation, this can naturally be achieved through the frequent use of the person's name and the presentation of current information in an informal way, such as: 'It is warm for February' or 'It is nice here in your own home'.

For others who are not at this level of ability, reality orientation may focus more on the raising of self-awareness. Sensory media may be used to stimulate engagement with the environment and the person may also respond to touch, gentle rocking movement and communication based on body language.

Being surrounded by familiar objects which can be used to stimulate an individual (such as family scrapbooks, photographs, memory books or boxes) can facilitate a very helpful and enjoyable communication opportunity.

By using this range of techniques and approaches, you or the person you support can improve function and reduce the symptoms of dementia through cognitive rehabilitation therapy and cognitive stimulation therapy.

A few thoughts on thinking

This chapter has focused on memory and techniques to support memory function in order to improve everyday function. One of the highest developed cognitive skills we have is thinking: the ability to reason and consider something.

There are two categories of thinking: concrete and abstract. Concrete thinking is the earlier skill that we learn and is specific to things, whereas abstract thinking is learned later as we mature and is the ability to have ideas and to reflect on events and relationships.

There are many examples of how we develop our abstract thinking, including the use of nursery stories (The Ugly Duckling, Little Red Riding Hood, Cinderella) that at face value (concrete) are stories of facts and events that happened to characters. However, the events and the characters are also metaphors for a deeper (abstract) meaning of how people in general can modify and control their behaviour. At older ages and higher levels of thinking, people can reach higher levels of abstraction. The process of learning to be an abstract thinker comes out of a discussion with an abstract thinker who is at a higher level than the learner.

Abstract language is said to include terms that refer to concepts, for example, 'justice' and 'freedom', as opposed to terms that refer to actual physical things, like 'chair' and 'car'. Abstract language also includes indirect uses of language, such as metaphors and figures of speech. For example, a concrete thinker would interpret 'People who live in glass houses should not throw stones' to refer literally to breakable panes of glass. An abstract thinker, in contrast, would understand that the figure of speech means that people who have faults of their own should not criticise others.

A symptom of the dementia that the individual is experiencing can be a loss of the ability to think in the abstract. This can be very frustrating to the person and to their family. There are no known 'exercises' in abstract thinking that have the effect of turning a concrete thinker into an abstract thinker across domains of content. Sometimes practice with brain teasers or maths and logic problems is suggested as a means to facilitate more abstract thinking. However, there is no evidence that this 'brain training' practice enhances abstract thinking in a generalisable way.

As abstract thinking and the use of abstract language is a highly developed and complex skill, it is best to ensure that concrete concepts and language are used to support under-standing, connection and the relationship with the person.

However, metaphors that were well understood before the symptoms of dementia arrived (e.g. 'Get lost') may be just as concrete and easy to understand as their literal equivalents ('Please leave'). Sometimes metaphors come to be so commonly used and easy to understand that we forget that they are metaphors, like 'He's a barrel of laughs'.

As with all the approaches outlined in this chapter, you will know the unique abilities and limitations of the individual and plan to support them based on this very individual approach.

This chapter has provided you with many ideas for how it is possible to apply cognitive approaches that overcome the impairment and restore functional skills. Table 6.1 below aims to give you a summary of these approaches; each should be applied to a functional goal that has been specifically identified. The solutions are therefore used within the context of the goal.

The process for applying the cognitive rehabilitation therapy restorative approach is:

1. **Identify a specific goal that is currently not possible because of a cognitive skill that is impaired.**

    For example:

    –   Orientation to time impairment will affect appointment keeping, attending a regular outing, eating a meal, taking medication, etc.

    –   Inability to recognise objects will affect eating a meal, taking medication, getting dressed, using the toilet, etc.

    –   Inability to follow through the sequence of steps in an activity will affect many activities of daily living.

2. **Set a SMART goal to achieve**

    For example:

    –   'In six weeks (date) I will know when to attend the hairdressers/eat my lunch/take my medication without asking others'

    –   'In six weeks (date) I will be able to recognise my meals and eat at least two-thirds of every dish'

-   'In six weeks (date) I will be able to find the bathroom without asking'

-   'In six weeks (date) I will be able to get dressed in the right order without any help'.

3. **Select from the cognitive rehabilitation therapy restorative strategies** in Table 6.1.

4. **Intensively practise the strategies** with four sessions a day for the first seven days and then review. If the goal is being achieved, gradually decrease the intensive practice sessions to once per day for the goal period that you have set.

   If the goal is not being met, or the technique is not being enjoyed, select a different strategy and start the goal over again.

Table 6.1. cognitive rehabilitation therapy restorative strategies

Memory impairment	Disability	Cognitive rehabilitation therapy restorative strategies
Memory encoding	Not aware of sensory cues to take in information	• Use of multi-modal sensory cues • Simplification of figure–background and noise–background environment • Prompting to attend to the sensory cues using alerting language and appropriate touch
Memory storage	No new memories formed (learning)	• Use of multi-modal sensory cues • Errorless learning • Expanding rehearsal • Chunking • Mnemonics
Memory recall	Inability to recall events, names, processes, etc.	• Mnemonics • Cueing • Prompting and fading of prompts

Now we are going to move onto the Rementia Plan where you will be able to see how these cognitive rehabilitation therapy restorative strategies can be brought together with the other cognitive rehabilitation approaches of good nutrition and hydration for physical well-being, good sleep, exercise and relationships for emotional well-being and helpful compensatory approaches for cognitive well-being. Together these approaches form a multi-therapeutic framework for you or the person you are supporting.

Chapter 7

Putting It All Together – The Rementia Plan

We have now reached the point of putting all of the factors that I have presented to you in this book into a multi-therapeutic plan. This plan is for the person who is living with the symptoms of dementia so the guidance in this chapter is addressed to that individual. Of course, the reader might also be the person who is supporting the individual, and in those cases the aim of this chapter is to encourage the supporting person to work in partnership with the individual: discussing their goals, what is meaningful to them and developing the Rementia Plan together.

Identifying your goals

The start of your own unique plan is to identify what is meaningful to you and then to set your own goals and techniques for how to achieve them.

This will possibly require a lifestyle change so you must decide if the 'end will justify the means' and that is why it is helpful to begin by identifying what is meaningful to you and setting those SMART goals to work towards.

To help you with this, here are seven steps that will support you.

Step 1: Identify what is important to you

Think about what would you look back on and regret not pursuing. What would you qualify as missed opportunities? These are likely to be the things that are most meaningful to you now, and the ones you should act upon today. Make a list of each of these experiences then follow the next steps to learn how to turn your priorities into meaningful goals.

These opportunities might include: spending time or staying connected with family or friends, keeping or regaining your independence in an everyday activity or continuing or starting a hobby or interest.

Step 2: List these opportunities as SMART goals

Now that you've worked out what is most important to you, it's time to turn these things into actionable goals.

To start, write down goals that you may want to consider for all of the opportunities that you have identified for yourself. Many of these will not make it to your Rementia Plan, and some will dramatically change before you commit to them. But for now, you're just putting it on paper.

Be sure to write down goals that are **S**pecific, **M**easurable, **A**chievable, **R**ealistic and **T**ime-specific (e.g. 'speak to my daughter once a week', 'go to the shops on my own every morning to collect the newspaper' or 'knit a blanket in time for the birth of my expected grandchild'). Make a long list – include at least 20 possible goals. Be spontaneous and don't allow yourself to be put off by what is getting in the way of you achieving these goals. You're not committing to anything yet!

Step 3: Vet your goals

The goals you are most likely to accomplish are the ones that have motivation built into them, meaning you don't have to talk yourself into doing them. We all have the deeply human need to direct our own lives, to learn and create new things, and to do better by ourselves and our world. The three elements of motivation are autonomy, mastery and purpose. So, in order to work out if a certain goal contains intrinsic motivation, ask yourself the following seven questions for each of your goals and write down the number of times you answer 'yes':

- Will this goal be satisfying for you to pursue and achieve?

- Is this goal something that you would do even if no one expects you to?

- Will the pursuit of this goal increase your ability to choose the things you do?

- Will the pursuit or accomplishment of this goal develop your skills and capabilities?

- Does this goal fit well with your other goals in life (i.e. it does not conflict with anything else you would like to accomplish)?

- Does the pursuit or accomplishment of this goal bring you close to others?

- Is this goal appropriate for your circumstances (like age, physical health, finances, etc.)?

Step 4: Select your most viable goals

Look at the goals for which you answered 'yes' the most times. It is probable that these goals will be the most fulfilling and the most possible for you to pursue. Choose two of these goals to get started. You can always return to your list later if you want to add more.

Step 5: Commit to your goals

Copy your selected goals to a fresh piece of paper and help yourself to have a clear mental image of each of them in your mind. To create this concrete vision of your goal, it's helpful to add an image to associate with each of your goals (e.g. a photo of your daughter, a picture that means 'freedom' to you or a baby wrapped in a knitted blanket).

Step 6: See the goals as the vehicle for your personal rehabilitation

At this stage, you've made your first steps of your Rementia Plan and we will look next at how you are going to address your physical, emotional and cognitive health in order to give you the best chance of achieving the goals.

The goals that you have chosen will support you to stick to your Rementia Plan and they will become the means for you to practise your cognitive rehabilitation techniques.

In daily routine, most people operate on autopilot (procedural memory), responding to triggers in their environment. You can take advantage of this by weaving the pursuit of your goals into your day-to-day life: add reminders in your calendar, place visual cues in opportunistic areas (e.g. place your knitting next to your armchair if you want to knit that blanket in the evening or place your jacket on the back of the dining room chair if you want to collect the newspaper after your breakfast).

Step 7: Look back and praise progress

When you're climbing up a hill, it can be discouraging to look up and realise how far away the top is. Instead, choose to look back and take pride in the ground you've already covered. Research by Dr Heidi Grant Halvorson (2010), a social psychologist, shows that people who 'focus on the prize' do not perform as well as those who are focused on their progress so far. Each time you feel discouraged, look back on your progress and give yourself a big pat on the back. You've earned it!

Getting started on your Rementia Plan

Now that you have clearly identified your personally meaningful goals, put them somewhere visible and get started on your Rementia Plan to support you in working towards them.

The Rementia Plan is set out in three tables, each one identifying action points and techniques for achieving these, with space for you to note your own methods and ideas. The tables are:

- **My Nutrition and Hydration Plan**

- **My Emotional Well-Being Plan**

- **My Cognitive Rehabilitation Therapy Plan**

I recommend that you address all three plans as together they will provide you with a multi-therapeutic systematic approach to improving your functional difficulties.

The tables are also available at www.jkp.com/voucher for personal use with this programme using the code HEYWUKE, or you are welcome to copy them from this book. They may not be reproduced for any other purposes without the permission of the publisher.

The Rementia Plan: Nutrition and hydration

I am not recommending any specific diet plans as you must investigate and decide for yourself if you wish to follow one. However, I am highly recommending that you look closely at the food that you eat and consider replacing foods which might be undermining your brain health with foodswhich could support it.

As I said in Chapter 4, if the food is good for your heart, it will also be good for your head. It is widely believed that the Mediterranean diet, or adopting some of the principles of the Paleo diet, are the best ways of achieving brain and body health through good nutrition, eating as naturally as possible by opting for grass-fed meats, fish, an abundance of fruit and veg and other wholefoods like nuts and seeds.

There is certainly a case for avoiding cereal grains, processed foods, low-fat dairy products, potatoes and fruit or veg that contain too much fructose. To begin with, this can seem daunting, as you wonder how to not eat bread, for example. I certainly would not recommend replacing your current bread with a gluten free alternative because it is likely to have even more additives and preservatives in it. Rather, look for ways of replacing bread altogether. I stopped eating bread several years ago and now find it surprisingly easy, but it does need a little forethought, especially if you are out and about as snacks and fast food are often centred around a sandwich or a bread bun. I opt for portable foods such as soups, salads, cheese, nuts and berries.

It could be easy to be drawn into a dogmatic approach to your diet and then it could be that your enjoyment of food becomes lowered. So, if I fancy an especially gorgeous-smelling home-made bread that is being served in a restaurant, I do have a small piece! Just let bread be a very occasional treat rather than the mainstay of your meals.

There are many good books and websites that will provide you with menu ideas, but following the actions in Table 7.1 will support you or the person you care for to eat well for your brain health. All pages marked with ↓ can be downloaded at www.jkp.com/voucher for personal use with this programme using the code HEYWUKE, but may not be reproduced for any other purposes without the permission of the publisher.

Table 7.1. My Nutrition and Hydration Plan

Action	Techniques	My personal notes
Avoid inflammatory foods	No gluten, cereal grains, processed foods or vegetable oils Eat wild lean meat, chicken, fish, green leafy vegetables, fruit, nuts, berries and honey	My favourite non-inflammatory foods:
Eat foods low in omega-6 fatty acids and high in omega-3 EFAs	No cereals, grains or vegetable oils Eat oily fish including salmon, sardines and mackerel	My favourite omega-3 EFA foods:
Maintain good cholesterol levels	Use extra virgin olive oil for cooking and dressings No foods containing trans fats such as doughnuts, cookies, crackers, muffins, pies and cakes No commercially fried foods and baked goods made with shortening or partially hydrogenated vegetable oils	My favourite oil:

cont.

Action	Techniques	My personal notes
Eat antioxidants	Eat green vegetables at every meal and for a snack (e.g. spinach in a smoothie) Eat berries as a dessert and keep the fruit bowl in sight and topped up	My favourite green vegetables: My favourite berries:
Keep blood sugars low	Ideally do not eat processed foods but if you do, check that it contains 5g or less of total sugar per 100g Switch biscuits and snacks to a handful of nuts (almonds, cashews or pistachios) Avoid high starch foods such as potatoes, parsnips and bananas	My favourite nuts and seeds:
Drink	Drink 1.2 litres a day	My favourite drinks:
Supplements	Consult a nutritional therapist for advice on: Omega-3 EFA and DHA Resveratrol Turmeric (curcumin) Probiotics alpha lipoic acid Vitamin D, C, E and beta carotene	My specified supplements:

Action	Techniques	My personal notes
Weight	Consult your GP or nutritional therapist for your optimum weight and body fat percentage	My weight target: My body fat percentage target:

The Rementia Plan: Emotional well-being

You have read in Chapter 5 that emotional well-being is critical to brain and body health and to functional ability and we explored the use of emotional intelligence and person-centred relationship techniques in order to reduce stress and support well-being.

In addition to these techniques, we also explored the importance of good sleep, exercise, relaxation and access to nature as restorative cognitive rehabilitation techniques.

Planning and following the actions in Table 7.2 will support you or the person you care for to experience greater emotional well-being, which will contribute to improved abilities.

Table 7.2. My Emotional Well-Being Plan

Action	Techniques	My personal notes
Exercise	Personalised daily routine of 30 minutes per day, 5 days per week	My passive exercises: Who is supporting me: My active exercises:
Sleep	Last meal is 3 hours before bedtime Sleep for 8 hours per night Drink 500ml of water on waking Breakfast 1 hour after waking Personalised sleep hygiene plan Improve nighttime breathing by avoiding alcohol, sleeping pills, and sedatives, especially before bedtime Open a bedroom window to let in clean air	My bedtime: My waking time: My getting to sleep routine:
Relaxation	Personalised daily routine of 30 minutes per day. Choose from activities such as meditation, mindfulness, yoga, pilates, music, gentle walking	My relaxation routine:

Action	Techniques	My personal notes
Social connection	Personalised plan for 60 minutes per week interaction with others	My social connection opportunities: Who is visiting me: Where I am going out: My hobbies: My interests: My history:
Fresh air	Personalised plan for a minimum of 5 minutes per day outdoors in natural environments	My access to nature and fresh air plan:
Anti-stress supplements	Consult your GP Consider decaffeinated or relaxation inducing herbal drinks	My specified anti-stress supplements: My favourite anti-stress drinks:

The Rementia Plan: Cognitive Rehabilitation Therapy

Tables 7.1 and 7.2 have enabled you to develop a personal Rementia Plan that will optimise the brain health of you or the person you care for by addressing lifestyle factors in a multi-therapeutic programme. This sets the foundation for now addressing the goals that you or the person has identified as meaningful to them.

You will recall that I described the Pool Activity Level (PAL) Instrument in Chapter 6 and that I have placed it in the Appendix for your use. When you are ready to begin your Cognitive Rehabilitation Therapy (CRT) Plan, complete the PAL Checklist in order to identify the PAL Level of Ability. This will support you to select from the four PAL Profiles provided so that you can understand how to present activities, objects and social interaction in ways that meet the person's needs.

In addition, your understanding of the person's PAL Level of Ability will support you to select the appropriate CRT Plan from the four provided.

The details of the approaches are provided in Chapter 6 where we explored how to select from the CRT restorative strategies in Table 6.1. In addition to the CRT Plans, I have also provided you with a sample of how each Plan will look at each of the four levels of ability for a specific goal. However, each one will be highly individual according to the goal and the difficulties that are getting in the way of achieving the goal.

Intensively practise the strategies with four sessions a day for the first seven days and then review how it is going. If the goal is being achieved, gradually decrease the intensive practice sessions to once per day for the goal period that you have set. Your minimum goal period should be six weeks but some goals, particularly if they are complex, can take longer. If there is no progress towards the goal, or the technique is not being enjoyed, select a different strategy and start the goal over again.

My Cognitive Rehabilitation Therapy Plan at a PAL Planned Activity Level of Ability

My goal:

_____

_____

_____

_____

Steps in my goal:

1. _____

2. _____

3. _____

4. _____

Techniques	My personal notes
Compensatory Memory aids Helpful environment	My memory aids are: _____ _____ My helpful environment for this goal is: _____ _____

Memory encoding Sensory cues Attention prompting	My sensory cues for this goal are: _____ _____ My sensory cues are in their usual, familiar place of: _____ _____ My attention is captured by reminding me where to look for: _____ _____
Memory storage Errorless learning Expanding rehearsal Chunking Mnemonics	My errorless learning will be supported in groups of three steps towards my goal My expanding rehearsal technique will be to acquire the factual information to achieve my goal My chunking of the factual information about my goal will be: _____ _____ My mnemonic to help me to store and recall the factual information about my goal will be: _____ _____
Memory recall Cueing Mnemonics Prompting and fading of prompts	My visual cues for recalling this factual information about my goal will be: _____ _____ My prompting to recall the factual information, including the mnemonic about my goal will be: _____ _____ My prompts will be faded as I learn this technique and demonstrate that I can use it safely

SAMPLE:

My Cognitive Therapy Rehabilitation Plan at a PAL Planned Activity Level of Ability

My goal:

I will visit the shop each morning to buy my daily newspaper.

Steps in my goal:

1. *I will always take my money and my key with me.*

2. *I will find my way to the shop and home again.*

3. *I will cross the road safely.*

Techniques	My personal notes
Compensatory Memory aids Helpful environment	My memory aids are: *Have a 'remember your bag' note on the door at eye height* My helpful environment for this goal is: *Keep my purse and key together in my bag next to the coat rack* *Cross the road at the pedestrian crossing*
Memory encoding Sensory cues Attention prompting	My sensory cues for this goal are: *My bag is red, my key and purse have a red pompom on them* My sensory cues are in their usual, familiar place of: *The coat rack, next to my black jacket* My attention is captured by reminding me where to look for: *My bag and for the pedestrian crossing*

Memory storage Errorless learning Expanding rehearsal Chunking Mnemonics	My errorless learning will be supported in groups of three steps towards my goal My expanding rehearsal technique will be to acquire the factual information to achieve my goal My chunking of the factual information about my goal will be: *Bring my bag – Cross at the crossing* *I will use 'Stop, look, listen and wait for the green man' when crossing* My mnemonic to help me to store and recall the factual information about my goal will be: *Be Cross*
Memory recall Cueing Mnemonics Prompting and fading of prompts	My visual cues for recalling this factual information about my goal will be: *My red bag; the note on the door; the pedestrian crossing* My prompting to recall the factual information, including the mnemonic about my goal will be: *'What do I have to take?'* *Supplementary prompt: 'Begins with B'* *'What colour is my bag?'* *'Where does my bag live?'* *'Where do I cross the road?'* My prompts will be faded as I learn this technique and demonstrate that I can use it safely

My Cognitive Rehabilitation Therapy Plan at a PAL Exploratory Activity Level of Ability

My goal:

_____

_____

Steps in my goal:

1. _____

2. _____

Techniques	My personal notes
Compensatory Memory aids Helpful environment	My memory aids are: _____ _____ My helpful environment for this goal is: _____ _____
Memory encoding Sensory cues Attention prompting	My sensory cues for this goal are: _____ _____ My sensory cues are in my line of sight in a 'workstation' next to my goal setting of: _____ _____ My attention is captured by pointing out to me what to look for: _____ _____

Memory storage	My errorless learning will be supported in pairs of two steps towards my goal
Errorless learning	My expanding rehearsal technique will be to acquire the factual and procedural information to achieve my goal
Expanding rehearsal	
Chunking	My chunking of the factual information about my goal will be:
Mnemonics	
	_____
	_____
	My mnemonic to help me to store and recall the factual information about my goal will be:
	_____
	_____
	My chunking of the procedural information about my goal will be:
	_____
	_____
Memory recall	My visual cues for recalling this factual information about my goal will be:
Cueing	
Mnemonics	_____
Prompting and fading of prompts	_____
	My prompting to recall the factual information, including the mnemonic about my goal will be:
	_____
	_____
	My prompting of the procedural information about my goal will be:
	_____
	_____
	My prompts will be faded as I learn this technique and demonstrate that I can use it safely

My Cognitive Rehabilitation Therapy Plan at a PAL Exploratory Activity Level of Ability

My goal:

I will knit a blanket in time for the birth of my expected grandchild.

Steps in my goal:

1. *I will have help to cast on and off each square that I will knit.*

2. *I will only use the knit stitch to make thirty-six 6x6 inch squares of three different colours.*

3. *I will have help to sew the squares together.*

Techniques	My personal notes
Compensatory Memory aids Helpful environment	My memory aids are: *Keep my bag of knitting on the table next to my armchair* *Have the instructions written on a page on my table* *A knitting row clicky counter* My helpful environment for this goal is: *Only have the colour ball and the square that I am knitting in my bag*
Memory encoding Sensory cues Attention prompting	My sensory cues for this goal are: *My knitting bag is next to a photo of my daughter and son-in-law* My sensory cues are in my line of sight in a 'workstation' next to my goal setting of: *On a table next to my armchair* My attention is captured by pointing out to me what to look for: *The photo of my daughter who is expecting a baby*

Memory storage Errorless learning Expanding rehearsal Chunking Mnemonics	My errorless learning will be supported in pairs of two steps towards my goal My expanding rehearsal technique will be to acquire the factual and procedural information to achieve my goal My chunking of the factual information about my goal will be: *Knit 36 lines for a square* *Press clicky at the end of each line* My mnemonic to help me to store and recall the factual information about my goal will be: *Knit 36, Clickety click* My chunking of the procedural information about my goal will be: *Practise clicking the counter before turning the needles for the next row*
Memory recall Cueing Mnemonics Prompting and fading of prompts	My visual cues for recalling this factual information about my goal will be: *A sample of a completed square on my table to measure against* *A colourful, fun clicky counter* My prompting to recall the factual information, including the mnemonic about my goal will be: *'Knit thirty - …?, Clickety - …?'* My prompting of the procedural information about my goal will be: *Hand on my forearm at the end of a line to raise awareness* My prompts will be faded as I learn this technique and demonstrate that I can use it safely

My Cognitive Rehabilitation Therapy Plan at a PAL Sensory Activity Level of Ability

My goal:

_____

_____

Steps in my goal:

1. _____

2. _____

Techniques	My personal notes
Compensatory Memory aids Helpful environment	My memory aids are: _____ _____ My helpful environment for this goal is: _____ _____
Memory encoding Sensory cues Attention prompting	My sensory cues for this goal are: _____ _____ My sensory cues are within my reach: _____ _____ My attention is captured by pointing to or by passing me the objects that I need for this goal: _____ _____

Memory storage Errorless learning Expanding rehearsal Chunking	My errorless learning will be supported in single steps towards my goal My expanding rehearsal technique will be to acquire the procedural information to achieve my goal My chunking of the procedural information about my goal will be to set a simple pattern of movement of: _____ _____
Memory recall Cueing Prompting and fading of prompts	My sensory cues for recalling this procedural information about my goal will be: _____ _____ My prompting to recall the procedural information about my goal will be: _____ _____ My prompts will be faded as I learn this technique and demonstrate that I can use it safely

SAMPLE:

My Cognitive Rehabilitation Therapy Plan at a PAL Sensory Activity Level of Ability

My goal:

I will make a fruit salad once a week.

Steps in my goal:

1. *I will select the fruit.*

2. *I will prepare the fruit.*

Techniques	My personal notes
Compensatory Memory aids Helpful environment	My memory aids are: *My helper will encourage me to participate in this goal activity* My helpful environment for this goal is: *I will sit at the kitchen table with the fruit, a bowl of water and a serving bowl and a dining knife*
Memory encoding Sensory cues Attention prompting	My sensory cues for this goal are: *My helper will share with me the enjoyment of tasting and smelling the fruit* My sensory cues are within my reach: *All items that I need are placed on the table and within reach* My attention is captured by pointing to or by passing me the objects that I need for this goal: *My helper will use words like 'Look!', 'Here, take this', to encourage me to reach for items* *My helper will hold out items to me just beyond my reach to encourage me to take them*

Memory storage	My errorless learning will be supported in single steps towards my goal
Errorless learning	
Expanding rehearsal	My expanding rehearsal technique will be to acquire the procedural information to achieve my goal
Chunking	My chunking of the procedural information about my goal will be to set a simple pattern of movement of:
	Reaching for each piece of fruit
	Washing it in the bowl of water
	Cutting it into pieces (if large)
	Placing it in the serving bowl
Memory recall	My sensory cues for recalling this procedural information about my goal will be:
Cueing	*Play the same music each time*
Prompting and fading of prompts	*Set the work table up in the same way each time*
	My prompting to recall the procedural information about my goal will be:
	Passing or indicating the next piece of fruit at completion of the previous piece
	Positive reinforcing statements and a sense of fun and enjoyment
	My prompts will be faded as I learn this technique and demonstrate that I can use it safely

My Cognitive Rehabilitation Therapy Plan at a PAL Reflex Activity Level of Ability

My goal:

_____

_____

Step in my goal:

1. _____

Techniques	My personal notes
Compensatory Helpful environment	My helpful environment for this goal is: _____ _____
Memory encoding Sensory cues Attention prompting	My sensory cues for this goal are: _____ _____ My sensory cues are connecting with my reflex zones: _____ _____ My attention is captured by stimulating my reflex responses: _____ _____
Memory storage Errorless learning Expanding rehearsal	My errorless learning will be supported in the single step that is my goal My expanding rehearsal technique will be to acquire the procedural information to achieve my goal

Memory recall	My sensory cues for recalling this procedural information about my goal will be:
Cueing	_____ _____

SAMPLE:

My Cognitive Rehabilitation Plan
at a PAL Reflex Activity Level of Ability

My goal:

I will respond positively to a hand massage three times a week.

Step in my goal:

1. *My helper will give me a hand massage using a lavender-scented hand cream.*

Techniques	My personal notes
Compensatory Helpful environment	My helpful environment for this goal is: *I will be seated in a comfortable chair* *My helper will be seated at right angles to me and at my eye level*
Memory encoding Sensory cues Attention prompting	My sensory cues for this goal are: *Relaxing music* *Firm and gentle touch* *Relaxing scent* My sensory cues are connecting with my reflex zones: *My helper will encourage my palmar grasp reflex by stroking the centre of my palm* My attention is captured by stimulating my reflex responses: *My helper will smile, nod and affirm my grasp reflex*

Memory storage Errorless learning Expanding rehearsal	My errorless learning will be supported in the single step that is my goal My expanding rehearsal technique will be to acquire the procedural information to achieve my goal: *I will be encouraged to hold out my hand for the massage* *I will be supported to raise my hand to my face to smell the cream and encouraged to do this independently*
Memory recall Cueing	My sensory cues for recalling this procedural information about my goal will be: *The same familiar music* *The same familiar hand cream* *The same familiar use of verbal prompts and reinforcing language*

Conclusion

Thank you for taking the time to read this book. I do hope that it will be helpful to you as a person who is living with the symptoms of dementia or someone who is helping a person to live well with the condition.

My aim has been to give as much information as I can from my own journey as a professional and as a family caregiver and, even in the course of writing this book, I have learned so much more while researching the facts and current knowledge and practice.

This is evidence of the exciting and promising time that we are now living through with regards to understanding the potential for people to live well with dementia and to not only experience psychological well-being because of positive relationships, but also to experience an improvement in functional ability because of improved brain health and use of the rehabilitation strategies that I have shared with you.

References and Reading List

Alzheimer's Association (2014) 'Alzheimer's disease facts and figures.' *Alzheimer's & Dementia 10*, 2.

Alzheimer's Disease International (2014) 'Nutrition and dementia.' Accessed on 23 April 2018 at www.alz.co.uk/sites/default/files/pdfs/nutrition-and-dementia.pdf.

Alzheimer's Society (2014) 'The Dementia-friendly Technology Charter.' Accessed on 23 April 2018 at www.alzheimers.org.uk/technologycharter.

Alzheimer's Society (2015) 'Science behind the headlines: How to reduce your risk and other popular topics.' Accessed on 23 May 2018 at https://www.alzheimers.org.uk/about-dementia/risk-factors-and-prevention?documentID=2211.

Alzheimer's Society (2017) 'The Memory Handbook.' Accessed on 23 April 2018 at www.alzheimers.org.uk/info/20113/publications_about_living_with_dementia/349/the_memory_handbook.

Aujla, R. (2017) *The Doctor's Kitchen.* London: HarperCollins.

Bahar-Fuchs, A., Clare, L. and Woods, R.T. (2013) 'Cognitive training and cognitive rehabilitation for mild to moderate Alzheimer's disease and vascular dementia.' *Cochrane Database of Systematic Reviews, Issue 6*, Art. No.: CD003260.

Ballard, C., Corbett, A., Orrell, M. *et al.* (2018) 'Impact of person-centred care training and person-centred activities on quality of life, agitation, and antipsychotic use in people with dementia living in nursing homes: A cluster-randomised controlled trial.' Accessed on 23 April 2018 at https://doi.org/10.1371/journal.pmed.1002500.

Barton, J. and Pretty J. (2010) 'What is the best dose of nature and green exercise for improving mental health? A multi-study analysis. *Environmental Science and Technology 44*, 10, 3947–3955.

Bjornebekk, A., Mathe, A.A. and Brene, S. (2005) 'The antidepressant effect of running is associated with increased hippocampal cell proliferation.' *International Journal of Neuropsychopharmacology 8*, 3, 357–368.

Bransford, J.D. and McCarrell, N.S. (1974) 'A Sketch of a Cognitive Approach to Comprehension: Some Thoughts about Understanding What It Means to Comprehend.' In W. Weimer and D. Palermo (eds) *Cognition and the Symbolic Processes.* New York: Lawrence Erlbaum.

Bredesen, D.E. (2014) 'Reversal of cognitive decline: A novel therapeutic program.' *Aging 6*, 9, 707–717.

Carroll, B.J. (2002) 'Ageing, stress and the brain.' *Novartis Foundation Symposium 242*, 26–36; discussion 36–45.

Cartwright, A. and Solloway, A. (2007) *Emotional intelligence: Activities for developing you and your business.* London: Routledge.

Chatterjee, R. (2017) *The 4 Pillar Plan. How to Relax, Eat, Move and Sleep Your Way to a Longer, Healthier Life.* London: Penguin.

Clare, L. (2008) *Neuropsychological Rehabilitation and People with Dementia.* Hove: Psychology Press.

Clare, L., Bayer, A., Burns, A. *et al.* (2013) 'Goal-oriented cognitive rehabilitation in early-stage dementia: Study protocol for a multi-centre single-blind randomised controlled trial (GREAT).' *Trials 14*, 152.

Clare, L., Linden, D.E., Woods, R.T. *et al.* (2010) 'Goal-oriented cognitive rehabilitation for people with early-stage Alzheimer's disease: A single-blind randomized controlled trial of clinical efficacy.' *American Journal of Geriatric Psychiatry 18*, 10, 928–939.

Clare, L. and Wilson, B.A. (2004) 'Memory rehabilitation for people with early-stage dementia: A single case comparison of four errorless learning methods.' *Zeitschrift für Gerontopsychologie und Psychiatrie 17*, 109–117.

Clare, L., Wilson, B.A., Breen, K. and Hodges, J.R. (1999) 'Errorless learning of face–name associations in early Alzheimer's disease.' *Neurocase 5*, 1, 37–46.

Clare, L., Wilson, B.A., Carter, G., Breen, K., Gosses, A. and Hodges, J.R. (2000) 'Intervening with everyday memory problems in dementia of Alzheimer type: An errorless learning approach.' *Journal of Clinical and Experimental Neuropsychology 22*, 1, 132–146.

Davis, D. (2012) 'Delirium increases the risk of developing new dementia eight-fold in older patients.' Accessed on 24 April 2018 at www.cam.ac.uk/research/news/delirium-increases-the-risk-of-developing-new-dementia-eight-fold-in-older-patients#sthash.3YonYRVQ.dpuf.

de Werd, M.M., Boelen, D., Rikkert, M. *et al.* (2013) 'Errorless learning of everyday tasks in people with dementia.' *Clinical Interventions in Aging 8*, 1177–1190.

Doidge, N. (n.d.) Norman Doidge speaking about brain plasticity. Accessed on 23 May 2018 at www.brainhq.com/brain-resources/brain-plasticity/brain-plasticity-luminaries/norman-doidge.

Doidge, N. (2007) *The Brain That Changes Itself: Stories of Personal Triumph from the Frontiers of Brain Science.* London: Penguin.

Ellison, J. (2017) 'A new angle on Alzheimer's disease: The inflammation connection.' Bright Focus Foundation. Accessed on 23 May 2018 at www.brightfocus.org/alzheimers/article/new-angle-alzheimers-disease-inflammation-connection.

Elwood, P., Galante, J., Pickering, J. *et al.* (2013) 'Healthy lifestyles reduce the incidence of chronic diseases and dementia: Evidence from the Caerphilly Cohort Study.' *PLoS ONE 8*, 12, e81877.

Giebel, C. and Challis, D. (2015) 'Translating cognitive and everyday activity deficits into cognitive interventions in mild dementia and mild cognitive impairment.' *International Journal of Geriatric Psychiatry 30*, 21–31.

Goleman, D. (1995) *Emotional Intelligence.* New York: Bantam.

Grant Halvorson, H. (2010) *Succeed: How We Can Reach Our Goals.* New York: Hudson Street Press.

Hadjivassilou, M. (1996) 'Does cryptic gluten sensitivity play a part in neurological illness?' *Lancet 347*, 8998, 369–371.

Hadjivassilou, M. (2002) 'Gluten sensitivity as a neurological illness.' *Neurology, Neurosurgery and Psychiatry 72*, 5, 560–563.

Harcombe, Z. (n.d.) 'We have got cholesterol completely wrong.' Accessed on 23 May 2018 at www.zoeharcombe.com/the-knowledge/we-have-got-cholesterol-completely-wrong.

Harcombe, Z., Baker, J.S., Cooper, S.M. *et al.* (2015) 'Evidence from randomised controlled trials did not support the introduction of dietary fat guidelines in 1977 and 1983: A systematic review and meta-analysis.' *Open Heart 2015*, 2. Accessed on 24 April 2018 at http://openheart.bmj.com/content/2/1/e000196.

Harding, A., Robinson, S.J., Crean, S. and Singhrao, S.K. (2017) 'Can better management of periodontal disease delay the onset and progression of Alzheimer's disease?' *Journal of Alzheimer's Disease 58*, 2, 337–348.

Heneka, M.T., Carson, M.J., El Khoury, J. *et al.* (2015) 'Neuroinflammation in Alzheimer's disease.' *The Lancet 14*, 388–405.

Holmes, C. (2018) 'Chronic stress as a risk factor for the development of Alzheimer's disease.' Accessed on 24 April 2018 at www.alzheimers.org.uk/info/20053/research_projects/650/chronic_stress_as_a_risk_factor_for_the_development_of_alzheimers_disease?_ga=2.118943370.2044843989.1520179653-20966 34716.1466867159.

Holzel, B., Carmody, J., Vangel, M. *et al.* (2011) 'Mindfulness practice leads to increases in regional brain gray matter density.' *Psychiatry Research 191*, 1, 36–43.

Kelly, M.E. and O'Sullivan, M. (2015) 'Strategies and Techniques for Cognitive Rehabilitation. Manual for Healthcare Professionals Working with Individuals with Cognitive Impairment.' Trinity College, Dublin. Accessed on 30 April 2018 at www.alzheimer.ie/Alzheimer/media/SiteMedia/Services/Cognitive-Rehabilitation-Manual.pdf.

Kim, E.J., Pellman, B. and Jeansok, J.K. (2015) 'Stress effects on the hippocampus: A critical review.' *Learning and Memory 22*, 9, 411–416.

King, K.A. (2014) *Getting REAL About Alzheimer's: Rementia through Engagement, Assistance, and Love.* Austin, TX: Plainview Press.

Kitwood, T. (1989) 'Brain, mind and dementia: With particular reference to Alzheimer's disease.' *Ageing and Society 9*, 1–15.

Kitwood, T. (1990) 'The dialectics of dementia: With particular reference to Alzheimer's disease.' *Ageing and Society 10*, 177–196.

Kitwood, T. (1997) *Dementia Reconsidered: The Person Comes First.* Maidenhead: Open University Press.

Kitwood, T. and Bredin, K. (1992) 'Toward a theory of dementia care: Personhood and wellbeing.' *Ageing and Society 12*, 3, 269–287.

Lazar, S. (2011) 'Neuroimaging: How meditation can reshape our brains.' Accessed on 30 April 2018 at https://www.youtube.com/watch?v=m8rRzTtP7Tc.

Ledoux, J.E. (2015) *Anxious: Using the Brain to Understand and Treat Fear and Anxiety.* London: Viking.

Luders, E., Cherbuin, N. and Kurth, F. (2015) 'Forever Young(er): Potential age-defying effects of long-term meditation on gray matter atrophy.' Frontiers in Psychology. Accessed on 24 April 2018 at www.frontiersin.org/articles/10.3389/fpsyg.2014.01551/full.

Macoir, J., Leroy, M., Routier, S. *et al.* (2014) 'Improving verb anomia in the semantic variant of primary progressive aphasia: The effectiveness of a semantic-phonological cueing treatment.' *Neurocase: The Basis of Cognition 21,* 4, 448–456.

Magri, F., Cravello, L., Barili, L. *et al.* (2005) 'Stress and dementia: The role of the hypothalamic-pituitary-adrenal axis.' *Aging Clinical and Experimental Research 18,* 2 167–170.

Molteni, R., Zheng, J.Q., Ying, Z. *et al.* (2004) 'Voluntary exercise increases axonal regeneration from sensory neurons.' *Proceedings of the National Academy of Sciences of the USA 101,* 22, 8473–8478.

National Institute of Neurological Disorders and Stroke (NINDS) (2017) 'Understanding sleep.' Accessed on 30 April 2018 at www.ninds.nih.gov/Disorders/Patient-Caregiver-Education/Understanding-Sleep.

NHS Choices (2017) 'Gum disease linked to increased risk of Alzheimer's disease.' Accessed on 30 April 2018 at www.nhs.uk/news/neurology/gum-disease-linked-increased-risk-alzheimers-disease.

Nolan, M., Brown, J., Davies, S. *et al.* (2006) 'The Senses Framework – improving care for older people through a relationship-centred approach.' Accessed on 24 April 2018 at http://shura.shu.ac.uk/280/1/PDF_Senses_Framework_Report.pdf.

Orrell, M., Yates, L., Leung, P. *et al.* (2017) 'The impact of individual Cognitive Stimulation Therapy (iCST) on cognition, quality of life, caregiver health, and family relationships in dementia: A randomised controlled trial.' *PLOS Medicine 14,* 3, e1002269.

PaleoLeap (2018) 'Why cholesterol is not bad.' Accessed on 30 April 2018 at https://paleoleap.com/cholesterol-is-not-bad.

Perlmutter, D. (2014) *Grain Brain: The Surprising Truth about Wheat, Carbs and Sugar – Your Brain's Silent Killers.* London: Yellow Kite Books, Hodder & Stoughton.

Perry, V.H., Anthony, D.C., Bolton, S.J. and Brown, H.C. (1997) 'The blood–brain barrier and the inflammatory response.' *Molecular Medicine Today 3*, 8, 335–341.

Pool, J. (2012) *The Pool Activity Level (PAL) Instrument for Occupational Profiling (4th edition)*. London: Jessica Kingsley Publishers.

Pool, J. (2015) *Alzheimer's Society Guide to the Dementia Care Environment ebook*. London: Alzheimer's Society. Available at www.amazon.co.uk/Alzheimers-Society-guide-dementia-environment-ebook/dp/B00U2T530Q.

Rogers, C.R. (1961) On becoming a person. Boston, MA: Houghton Mifflin.

Sixsmith, A. (1993) 'Rementia – Challenging the limits of dementia care.' *International Journal of Geriatric Psychiatry 8*, 12, 993–1000.

Smyth, C. (2017) 'Gum disease sufferers 70% more likely to get dementia.' *The Times*, 22 August.

Spaemann, R. (2006) *Persons: The Difference between 'Someone' and 'Something'*, trans. O. O'Donovan. Oxford: Oxford University Press.

Strøm-Tejsen, P., Zukowska, D., Wargocki, P. *et al.* (2015) 'The effects of bedroom air quality on sleep and next-day performance.' *Indoor Air 26*, 5, 679–686.

UK Government (2015) 'When a mental health condition becomes a disability.' Accessed on 24 April 2018 at www.gov.uk/when-mental-health-condition-becomes-disability.

Vauzoura, D., Camprubi-Robles, M., Miquel-Kergoat, S. *et al.* (2017) 'Nutrition for the ageing brain: Towards evidence for an optimal diet.' *Ageing Research Reviews 35*, 222–240.

Wade, D.T. (2009) 'Goal setting in rehabilitation: An overview of what, why and how.' *Clinical Rehabilitation 23*, 291–295

Wenborn, J., Challis, D., Pool, J. *et al.* (2008) 'Assessing the validity and reliability of the Pool Activity Level (PAL) Checklist for use with older people with dementia.' *Aging and Mental Health 12*, 2, 202–211.

Wilson, L. (2013) 'Preventing malnutrition in later life.' Malnutrition Task Force. International Longevity Centre. Accessed on 24 April 2018 at www.malnutritiontaskforce.org.uk.

Woodall, J. (2013) '20 Minute Guided Mindfulness Exercise.' Accessed on 24 April 2018 at www.youtube.com/watch?v=thYoV-MCVs0.

Woods, B., Aguirre, E., Spector, A.E. and Orrell, M. (2011) 'Cognitive stimulation to improve cognitive functioning in people with dementia.' *Cochrane Database of Systematic Reviews 2005*, 4. Art. No.: CD005562.

Appendix: The Pool Activity Level (PAL) Instrument

This copy of the PAL Instrument, including the Checklist and the Profile, may be photocopied for your manual use for yourself or with the people for whom you care. All pages marked with ⬇ can be downloaded at www.jkp.com/ voucher using the code HEYWUKE for personal use with this programme, but may not be reproduced for any other purposes without the permission of the publisher.

Completing the PAL Checklist

Consider how you or the person with cognitive impairment generally functions when carrying out the activities described in the Checklist. If you are completing this for yourself, it will be helpful to discuss it with others who are close to you and who are able to observe your abilities in the described functions as, like us all, you may not be aware of or have the insight into all of your own capabilities and limitations. If you are completing the Checklist for another person and you are unsure about their abilities, observe the person in the situations over a period of two weeks. If the person lives in a group setting, such as a home, you might need to ask other caregivers for their observations too.

For each activity, the statements refer to a different level of ability. Thinking of the last two weeks, tick the statement that represents the person's ability in each activity. There should be only one tick for each activity. If in doubt about which statement to tick, choose the level of ability that represents their average performance over the last two weeks. Make sure you tick only one statement for each of the activities.

Sometimes the person might not be carrying out an activity to their full ability; consider the questions in the context of what they **can** do rather than only in the context of what they **are** currently doing.

Interpreting the Checklist

People do not fit neatly into boxes, and the PAL Instrument is designed to describe people in simple terms so that it is widely applicable. Add up the number of ticks for each activity level and enter the number in the total box at the end of the Checklist. You should find that there is a majority of ticks in one of the levels. This indicates which Activity Profile to select. If the number of ticks is almost evenly divided between two activity levels, assume that the person is currently functioning at the lower level of ability for the purpose of selecting the Activity Profile, but ensure that the person has an opportunity to move into the higher level of ability.

Using the Activity Profile

This is a general description of the environment in which the person is likely to best engage in activities. The information in the Activity Profile supports your development of the Rementia Plan.

Pool Activity Level (PAL) Checklist

Name: _____ Date: _____

Completed by: _____

Activity Level indicated:

Fill in after completing the checklist

Ensure you are familiar with the instructions before completion

Completing the Checklist	Key
• Thinking of the last 2 weeks, tick the statement that represents the person's ability in each section.	P = Planned level of ability
• If in doubt about which statement to tick, choose the level of ability that represents their average performance over the last 2 weeks.	E = Exploratory level of ability S = Sensory level of ability
• There should only be ONE TICK for each section.	
• You must tick one statement for each section.	R = Reflex level of ability
• Total the ticks at the bottom of each column at the end of the form.	

1. Bathing/Washing	P	E	S	R
• Can bathe/wash independently, sometimes with a little help to start				
• Needs soap put on flannel and one step at a time directions to wash				
• Mainly relies on others but will wipe own face and hands if encouraged				
• Totally dependent and needs full assistance to wash or bathe				

cont.

2. Getting dressed	P	E	S	R
• Plans what to wear, selects own clothing from the cupboards; dresses in correct order	☐			
• Needs help to plan what to wear but recognises items and how to wear them; needs help with order of dressing		☐		
• Needs help to plan and with order of dressing but can carry out small activities if someone directs each step			☐	
• Totally dependent on someone to plan, sequence and complete dressing; may move limbs to assist				☐

3. Eating	P	E	S	R
• Eats independently and using the correct cutlery	☐			
• Eats using a spoon and/or needs food to be cut up into small pieces		☐		
• Only uses fingers to eat food			☐	
• Relies on others to be fed				☐

4. Contact with others	P	E	S	R
• Initiates social contact and responds to the needs of others	☐			
• Aware of others and will seek interaction but may be more concerned with own needs		☐		
• Aware of others but waits for others to make the first social contact			☐	
• May not show an awareness of the presence of others unless in direct physical contact				☐

5. Groupwork skills	P	E	S	R
• Engages with others in a group activity; can take turns with the activity/tools	☐			
• Occasionally engages with others in a group, moving in and out of the group		☐		
• Aware of others in the group and will work alongside others although tends to focus on own activity			☐	
• Does not show awareness of others in the group unless close one-to-one attention is experienced				☐

6. Communication skills	P	E	S	R
• Is aware of appropriate interaction, can chat coherently and is able to use complex language skills		▓	▓	▓
• Language may be inappropriate and may not always be coherent but can use simple language skills and body language	▓		▓	▓
• Responses to verbal interaction may be mainly through body language; comprehension is limited	▓	▓		▓
• Can only respond to direct physical contact from others through touch, eye contact or facial expression	▓	▓	▓	

7. Practical activities (craft, domestic chores, gardening)	P	E	S	R
• Can plan to carry out an activity, hold the goal in mind and work through a familiar sequence; may need help solving problems		▓	▓	▓
• More interested in the making or doing than the end result, needs prompting to remember purpose, can get distracted	▓		▓	▓
• Activities need to be broken down and presented one step at a time, multi-sensory stimulation can help hold the attention	▓	▓		▓
• Unable to 'do' activities, but responds to the close contact of others and experiencing physical sensations	▓	▓	▓	

8. Use of objects	P	E	S	R
• Plans to use and looks for objects that are not visible; may struggle if objects are not in usual/familiar places (e.g. toiletries in a bathroom cupboard)		▓	▓	▓
• Selects objects appropriately only if in view (e.g. toiletries on a shelf next to the wash basin)	▓		▓	▓
• Randomly uses objects as chances upon them; may use appropriately	▓	▓		▓
• May grip objects when placed in the hand but will not attempt to use them	▓	▓	▓	

cont.

9. Looking at a newspaper/magazine	P	E	S	R
• Comprehends and shows interest in the content; turns the pages and looks at headlines and pictures				
• Turns the pages randomly, only attending to items pointed out by others				
• Will hold and may feel the paper, but will not turn the pages unless directed and will not show interest in the content				
• May grip the paper if it is placed in the hand but may not be able to release the grip or may not take hold of the paper				
N.B. If the totals are evenly divided between activity levels, assume that the person is at the lower level but has the potential to move into the higher level				
Totals				

The Activity Level identified for this person is:

_____

Transfer this information to the front of the form

Now use the relevant Pool Activity Level (PAL) Profile to assist you to plan how you will help the person with their Rementia Plan

Pool Activity Level (PAL) Profile ©
Planned Activity Level of Ability

Name: _____ Date: _____

Likely abilities

- Can explore different ways of carrying out an activity.

- Can work towards completing an activity with a tangible result.

- Can look in obvious places for any equipment.

Likely limitations

- May not be able to solve problems that arise.

- May not be able to understand complex sentences.

- May not search beyond the usual places for equipment.

Helper's role

- To enable the person to take control of the activity and master the steps involved.

- To encourage the person to initiate social interactions.

- To solve problems as they arise.

Using the PAL Profile to support the person

Position of objects	Ensure that equipment and materials are in their usual, familiar places.
Verbal directions	Explain activity using short sentences by avoiding using connecting phrases such as 'and', 'but', 'therefore' or 'if'. Allow time for a response. Repeat the directions if the person is struggling to recall the guidance. Encourage the person to solve problems encountered through gentle prompts.
Demonstrated directions	Show the person how to avoid possible errors. If problems cannot be solved independently then demonstrate the solution. Encourage them to then copy.
Working with others	The person is able to make the first contact and should be encouraged and be given opportunity to initiate social contact.
Activity characteristics	There is a goal or end product, with a set process, or 'recipe', to achieve it.

Pool Activity Level (PAL) Profile ©
Exploratory Activity Level of Ability

Name: _____ Date: _____

Likely abilities

- Can carry out very familiar activities in familiar surroundings.

- Enjoys the experience of doing an activity more than the end result.

- Can carry out more complex activities if they are broken down into two to three step stages.

Likely limitations

- May not have an end result in mind when starts an activity.

- May not recognise when the activity is completed.

- Relies on cues such as diaries, newspaper, lists and labels.

Helper's role

- To enable the person to experience the sensation of doing the activity rather than focusing on the end result.

- To break the activity into manageable chunks.

- To keep directions simple and understandable.

- To approach and make first contact as it is rarely initiated by the person.

Using the PAL Profile to support the person

Position of objects	Ensure that equipment and materials are in the line of vision.
Verbal directions	Explain activity using short simple sentences. Avoid using connecting phrases such as 'and', 'but' or 'therefore'. Also avoid using prepositions such as 'in', 'by' or 'for'. Repeat the directions if the person is struggling to recall the guidance.
Demonstrated directions	Break the activity into two to three steps at a time.
Working with others	Others must approach the person and make the first contact.
Activity characteristics	There is no pressure to perform to a set of rules, or to achieve an end result. There is an element of creativity and spontaneity.

Pool Activity Level (PAL) Profile ©
Sensory Activity Level of Ability

Name: _____ Date: _____

Likely abilities

- Is likely to be responding to bodily sensations.

- Can be guided to carry out single step activities.

- Can carry out more complex activities if they are broken down into one step at a time.

Likely limitations

- May not have any conscious plan to carry out a movement to achieve a particular end result.

- May be relying on others to make social contact.

Helper's role

- To enable the person to experience the effect of the activity on their senses

- To break the activity into one step at a time.

- To keep directions simple and understandable.

- To approach and make the first contact with the person.

Using the PAL Profile to support the person

Position of objects	Ensure that the person becomes aware of equipment and materials by making bodily contact.
Verbal directions	Limit requests to carry out actions to the naming of the action and of the object involved, e.g. 'lift your arm', 'hold the brush'.
Demonstrated directions	Demonstrate to the person the action on the object. Break the activity down into one step at a time.
Working with others	Others must approach the person and make the first contact. Use touch and the person's name to sustain the social contact.
Activity characteristics	The activity is used as an opportunity for a sensory experience. This may be multi-sensory. Repetitive actions are appropriate.

Pool Activity Level (PAL) Profile ©
Reflex Activity Level of Ability

Name: _____ Date: _____

Likely abilities

- Can make reflex responses to direct sensory stimulation.

- Direct sensory stimulation can increase awareness of self, and others.

- May respond to social engagement through the use of body language.

Likely limitations

- May not be aware of the surrounding environment or even their own body.

- May have difficulty organising the multiple sensations that are being experienced.

- May become agitated in an environment that is over-stimulating.

Helper's role

- To enable the person to be more aware of themselves.

- To arouse the person to be more aware of their surroundings.

- To engage with the person through direct sensory stimulation.

- To monitor the environment and reduce multiple stimuli, loud noises and background sounds.

Using the PAL Profile to support the person

Position of objects	Direct stimuli to the area of body being targeted, e.g. stroke the person's arm before placing it in a sleeve. Use light across the person's field of vision to encourage eye movement.
Verbal directions	Limit spoken directions to movement directions, e.g. 'Lift', 'Hold', 'Open'. Use a warm, reassuring tone and adapt volume to establish a connection with the person.
Demonstrated directions	Guide movements by touching the relevant body part.
Working with others	Maintain eye contact, make maximum use of facial expression, gestures and body posture for a non-verbal conversation. Use social actions which can be imitated, e.g. smiling, waving, shaking hands.
Activity characteristics	The activity focuses on a single sensation: touch, smell, sound, sight, taste.

Subject Index

Tables are identified by **bold** type

Author Index